PENNSYLVANIA COLLEGE OF TECHNOLOGY LIBR

5 0608 01083172 4

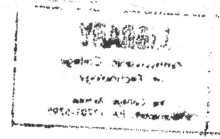

Manual of Retinal Surgery

Date Due

APR 16 2002			
FEB 2 3 2003			
	DISCARDED		

BRODART, CO.   Cat. No. 23-233-003   Printed in U.S.A.

D1299845

LIBRARY

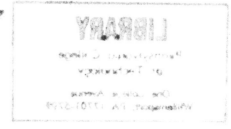

LIBRARY
Pennsylvania College
of Technology
One College Avenue
Williamsport, PA 17701-5799

Manual of Retinal Surgery

Second Edition

Edited by

Andrew J. Packer, M.D.

Associate Clinical Professor of Surgery, Department of Ophthalmology, University of Connecticut School of Medicine, Farmington; Senior Surgeon, Department of Ophthalmology, Hartford Hospital, Hartford

Foreword by

Thomas M. Aaberg, Sr., M.D.

F. Phinizy Calhoun, Sr., Professor and Chairman, Department of Ophthalmology, Emory University School of Medicine, Atlanta

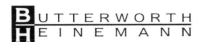

Boston   Oxford   Auckland   Johannesburg   Melbourne   New Delhi

LIBRARY
Pennsylvania College
of Technology
One College Avenue
Williamsport, PA 17701-5799

SEP 07

Copyright © 2001 by Butterworth–Heinemann

 A member of the Reed Elsevier group

All rights reserved.

No part of this publication may be reproduced, stored in a retrieval system, or transmitted in any form or by any means, electronic, mechanical, photocopying, recording, or otherwise, without the prior written permission of the publisher.

Every effort has been made to ensure that the drug dosage schedules within this text are accurate and conform to standards accepted at time of publication. However, as treatment recommendations vary in the light of continuing research and clinical experience, the reader is advised to verify drug dosage schedules herein with information found on product information sheets. This is especially true in cases of new or infrequently used drugs.

 Recognizing the importance of preserving what has been written, Butterworth–Heinemann prints its books on acid-free paper whenever possible.

AMERICAN FORESTS
GLOBAL ReLEAF 2000   Butterworth–Heinemann supports the efforts of American Forests and the Global ReLeaf program in its campaign for the betterment of trees, forests, and our environment.

Library of Congress Cataloging-in-Publication Data

Manual of retinal surgery / edited by Andrew J. Packer ; with a foreword by Thomas M. Aaberg.—2nd ed.
    p. ; cm.
  Includes bibliographical references and index.
  ISBN 0-7506-7106-8 (alk. paper)
  1. Retina—Surgery—Handbooks, manuals, etc. I. Packer, Andrew J.
  [DNLM: 1. Retina—surgery. WW 270 M294 2001]
 RE551 .M36 2001
 617.7'35059—dc21

00-045465

British Library Cataloguing-in-Publication Data
A catalogue record for this book is available from the British Library.

The publisher offers special discounts on bulk orders of this book.
For information, please contact:

Manager of Special Sales
Butterworth–Heinemann
225 Wildwood Avenue
Woburn, MA 01801-2041
Tel: 781-904-2500
Fax: 781-904-2620

For information on all Butterworth–Heinemann publications available, contact our World Wide Web home page at: http://www.bh.com

10 9 8 7 6 5 4 3 2 1

Printed in the United States of America

Cover art by Laurel C. Lhowe.

Contents

Contributing Authors   vii

Foreword by Thomas M. Aaberg, Sr.   ix

Preface   xi

1. Anatomy and General Considerations   1
   Andrew J. Packer

2. Preoperative Evaluation of the Retinal Detachment Patient   5
   Stanley Chang

3. Preoperative Ophthalmic Echography and Electrophysiology   11
   Robert E. Leonard II and Dwain G. Fuller

4. Laser Photocoagulation and Cryopexy of Retinal Breaks   23
   David W. Parke II

5. Pneumatic Retinopexy   33
   Paul E. Tornambe

6. Anesthesia for Vitreoretinal Surgery   43
   W. Sanderson Grizzard

7. Scleral Buckling Surgery (Cryopexy and Explants)   55
   Andrew J. Packer

8. Posterior Segment Vitrectomy   69
   Gary W. Abrams and Jane C. Werner

9. Macular Hole Surgery   105
   Lawrence S. Morse, Robert T. Wendel, and Peter T. Yip

10. Complications and Postoperative Management   119
    Mark S. Blumenkranz

Index   131

Contributing Authors

Gary W. Abrams, M.D.
Professor and Chairman of Ophthalmology, Kresge Eye Institute, Wayne State University, Detroit

Mark S. Blumenkranz, M.D.
Professor and Chairman of Ophthalmology, Stanford University School of Medicine, and Stanford Medical Center, Stanford, California

Stanley Chang, M.D.
Professor and Chairman of Ophthalmology, Columbia University, New York; Director, Edward S. Harkness Eye Institute, New York Presbyterian Hospital, New York

Dwain G. Fuller, M.D.
Clinical Associate Professor and former Chairman of Ophthalmology, Southern Medical School, Dallas

W. Sanderson Grizzard, M.D.
President and Chief Operating Officer, Retina Associates of Florida, Tampa

Robert E. Leonard II, M.D.
Clinical Assistant Professor of Ophthalmology, Texas Tech University, Lubbock; Attending Physician of Ophthalmology, Covenant Health Care System, Lubbock

Lawrence S. Morse, M.D., Ph.D.
Professor of Ophthalmology, University of California—Davis, Sacramento

Andrew J. Packer, M.D.
Associate Clinical Professor of Surgery, Department of Ophthalmology, University of Connecticut School of Medicine, Farmington; Senior Surgeon, Department of Ophthalmology, Hartford Hospital, Hartford

David W. Parke II, M.D.
Edward L. Gaylord Professor and Chairman of Ophthalmology, University of Oklahoma College of Medicine, Oklahoma City; President, Dean A. McGee Eye Institute, Oklahoma City

Paul E. Tornambe, M.D.
Director, Retina Research Foundation of San Diego, California; Scripp Memorial Hospital, Mericose Eye Institute, La Jolla, California

Robert T. Wendel, M.D.
Clinical Faculty of Ophthalmology, University of California—Davis, Sacramento; Retinal Consultants, Private Practice, Sacramento

Jane C. Werner, M.D.
Retinal Specialists, Ann Arbor, Michigan

Peter T. Yip, B.A.
Medical Student and Pre-Doctoral Research Fellow of Ophthalmology, University of California—Davis, Sacramento

Foreword

A manual is a book that helps its readers understand and perform a technique. Alternatively, it can be defined as a book limited to the important facts and necessary instructions to accomplish a task. Both definitions ably describe the *Manual of Retinal Surgery.*

Dr. Andrew J. Packer and his colleagues have updated and expanded the topics of this edition while retaining the concise technique descriptions that will prove remarkably useful for students of ophthalmology as well as practicing ophthalmologists who wish to bring their understanding of current vitreoretinal techniques to current frontiers. Little time is spent on esoteric topics; instead each chapter succinctly presents the basic information needed to understand the principles and techniques. In the decade since the previous edition, new indications for vitrectomy have been defined, hence the expansion of Chapter 8 on posterior segment vitrectomy and the new chapter on macular hole surgery. While presenting the current accepted indications for procedures that have passed the test of peer review, it is not all-inclusive of vitrectomy indications proposed by small or anecdotal reports. This is not a compendium of reference material. Indeed, each chapter lists only a limited number of pertinent recent references and classic historical references. The book is intended to communicate basic principles and does an admirable job of accomplishing that task.

Preoperative evaluation to detect the location in a detached retina of the causative retinal holes is well described, as are adjunctive ultrasound and electrophysiologic tests necessary to determine the nature of retinal detachments when opacities of the media are present.

The chapter on selection of treatment modalities is useful when considering the perpetual question of whether laser therapy or cryopexy should be used for treatment of symptomatic retinal tears, as well as for its descriptions of the actual methods of both techniques. A discussion of the contemporarily popular pneumatic retinopexy follows, with detailed instruction of the use of gas tamponade of retinal breaks. With now a decade more of experience with the pneumatic technique, the author concludes with a personal philosophical justification for the procedure that readers will find interesting and provocative.

All surgeons involved in retinal procedures will find the chapter on techniques of local anesthesia and indications for general anesthesia to be useful. The subsequent chapter on the technique of explant scleral buckling surgery is extremely detailed and certainly serves as the intended "manual" for both beginning and advanced retinal surgeons.

The chapter on complicated retinal detachment requiring posterior vitrectomy has been expanded to include current indications and techniques of subretinal surgery for choroidal neovascular membranes as well as foveal translocation. Finally, as the indications for surgical intervention have grown, so have the complications that can occur during and subsequent to retinal detachment surgery, as described in the last chapter.

I recommend this book to ophthalmologists at all levels of training who may wish to refine or revise their techniques or learn alternative ways to accomplish the repair of retinal detachment.

Thomas M. Aaberg, Sr., M.D.

Preface

The purpose of this manual is to provide the reader with a straightforward, practical guide to retinal surgery. It is not designed to provide a complete compendium on the topic but rather an up-to-date, reasonable approach. This second edition provides current indications as well as technical updates for the surgical procedures and includes a new chapter on macular hole surgery. Many of the personal preferences presented in this manual are intended to serve as suggestions for the surgeon who is looking to develop or modify his approach to retinal detachment surgery. The reader must keep in mind that there are many valid alternative techniques that are not covered. The suggested readings at the conclusion of each chapter will enable readers to cover selected areas in greater depth and will also acquaint them with valid alternative techniques. It is hoped that residents and beginning vitreoretinal fellows will use this manual as a starting point to help formulate their approach to retinal detachment surgery, and that practicing ophthalmologists will find some useful clinical "pearls" that will assist them in modifying their own individual approach.

I would like to acknowledge and thank Laurel C. Lhowe and Jerry Sewell, who created the wonderful illustrations for this edition.

Andrew J. Packer, M.D.

Manual of Retinal Surgery

1

Anatomy and General Considerations

Andrew J. Packer

Rhegmatogenous retinal detachments are caused by retinal breaks, which in most cases result from vitreoretinal traction. Fluid accumulates between the sensory retina and the retinal pigment epithelium (RPE). Closing (or sealing) the retinal break is synonymous with repairing (or preventing) a rhegmatogenous retinal detachment, assuming that the vitreoretinal traction has been relieved. Understanding the anatomic and physiologic principles of the posterior segment is essential to formulating appropriate treatment for retinal breaks and retinal detachments.

Retinal Anatomy

The retina is a thin, transparent tissue that lines the posterior two-thirds of the globe. The retina varies in thickness from 0.13 mm (in the center of the fovea) to 0.55 mm (at the margin of the anatomic fovea). It extends from the optic nerve posteriorly to the ora serrata anteriorly (which approximates the line of recti muscle insertion). Photoreceptors (rods and cones) are connected to neuronal pathways terminating in nonmyelinated fibers that form the optic nerve. The inner two-thirds of the retina are nourished by the retinal circulation; the outer one-third of the retina is nourished by the choroidal circulation, a high flow circulation that also serves as the cooling system for the eye (Figure 1-1).

The vortex veins, which are readily visible through the retina, are important landmarks because they exit through the sclera, approximately 3 mm posterior to the equator. There are usually four to six vortex veins, and they are frequently found near the 1, 5, 7, and 11 o'clock meridians (Figure 1-2). Ciliary nerves also serve as landmarks.

The anatomic macula is defined as the posterior portion of the retina containing two or more layers of ganglion cells. It measures from 5.5–7.5 mm in diameter and is centered approximately 4 mm temporal to and 0.8 mm inferior to the center of the optic disc. Clinically, this region is often referred to as the *posterior pole*.

The anatomic fovea is a depression in the inner retinal surface in the center of the macula measuring 1.5 mm in diameter. The anatomic fovea is commonly referred to clinically as the macula. On the external surface of the globe, it is centered 1 mm medial to and 1 mm above the posterior border of the inferior oblique insertion.

The RPE, a single layer of pigmented epithelium, is located external to the sensory retina, and the choroid is located external to the RPE. The choriocapillaris (the capillary bed of the choroid) is located adjacent to the RPE, allowing access to the outer retina, which it nourishes (Figure 1-1). The retina, the RPE, and the choroid are mechanically supported by the sclera, which varies in thickness from 0.3 mm (just posterior to the insertions of the

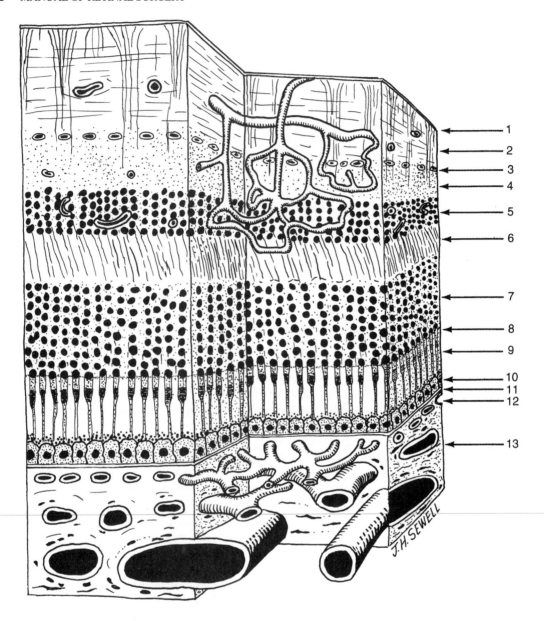

1. Inner Limiting Membrane
2. Nerve Fiber Layer
3. Ganglion Layer
4. Inner Plexiform Layer
5. Inner Nuclear Layer
6. Outer Plexiform Layer
7. Outer Nuclear Layer

8. External Limiting Membrane
9. Photoreceptor Inner and Outer Segments
10. Pigment Epithelium
11. Bruch's Membrane
12. Choriocapillaris
13. Choroid

Figure 1-1. Retinal anatomy. (Modified with permission from Bargmann W. *Histologie und Mikroscopische Anatomie des Menschen*. 6th ed. Georg Thieme, Stuttgart; 1967.)

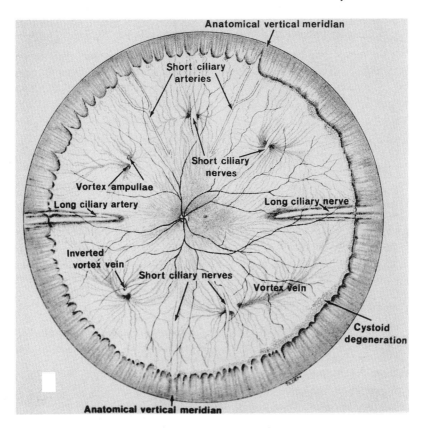

Figure 1-2. Retinal landmarks. (Reprinted with permission from Rutnin U, Schepens CL. Fundus appearance in normal eyes. *Am J Ophthalmol* 1967;64:824.)

recti muscles) to greater than 1.0 mm (near the posterior pole). Abnormally thin, blue-appearing areas of sclera called staphylomata can be found in eyes with retinal detachments. Narrow, radially oriented scleral dehiscences are also seen.

The Vitreous

The vitreous occupies a volume of approximately 4 cc in an emmetropic eye. It is firmly attached in a 2- to 4-mm-wide band at the ora serrata (the vitreous base) and is less tightly bound posteriorly (at the optic nerve, the macula, and along retinal blood vessels). It can also form abnormal focal adhesions, especially around areas of lattice degeneration and regions of chorioretinal scarring. The vitreous is a complex gel composed of collagen fibrils and hyaluronic acid. As a result of degenerative changes (as well as trauma, hemorrhage, and inflammatory changes), the vitreous may separate from the neu-

rosensory retina starting posteriorly; this is called a posterior vitreous separation (PVS) or posterior vitreous detachment (PVD). In the normal eye, the degeneration involves formation of large liquid cavities within the vitreous body. Contents of the liquefied cavities extrude posteriorly through defects in the posterior hyaloid, which then separates and collapses anteriorly.

In most cases, a PVD should be considered a normal process of an aging eye, present clinically in up to 65% of patients over 65 years of age. As the vitreous separates posteriorly, it remains firmly attached to the retina at the vitreous base. This places anteroposterior traction on any focal areas of vitreoretinal adhesion, which can lead to a retinal break as the vitreous is pulled anteriorly (Figure 1-3). Retinal breaks that are specifically caused by vitreous traction are referred to as *retinal tears* (also called "flap" tears or "horseshoe" tears because of the U-shaped defect that typically occurs). Ongoing traction on the anterior edge of a horseshoe tear will

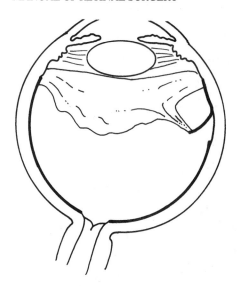

Figure 1-3. Posterior vitreous separation with focal vitreo-retinal adhesion causing a retinal tear.

tend to open the tear and encourage accumulation of subretinal fluid. If a section of retina is completely torn from the retinal surface, an operculated tear results. The round operculum can usually be seen hovering over the retinal defect. Since operculated tears are not affected by ongoing vitreoretinal traction, they are in general less likely to allow accumulation of subretinal fluid once opposed to the RPE. Retinal breaks located within the vitreous base are also not subject to ongoing tractional forces and are, therefore, less likely to go on to retinal detachment.

Several forces tend to promote attachment of the sensory retina to the underlying RPE; these include the RPE pump (creating negative pressure in the subretinal space), intercellular mucopolysaccharide "glue" between the RPE and the sensory retina, and possibly interdigitation of the RPE cell processes and the rods and cones of the sensory retina.

Factors that tend to promote retinal detachment, other than vitreoretinal traction, include the size of the retinal break and the dynamics of fluid currents within the vitreous cavity.

Suggested Reading

Hilton GF, McLean JB, Brinton DA. *Retinal Detachment: Principles and Practice.* 2nd ed. San Francisco: American Academy of Ophthalmology; 1995.

Jones LT, Reeh MJ, Wirtschafter JD. Ophthalmic anatomy. In: *American Academy of Ophthalmology Manual.* San Francisco: American Academy of Ophthalmology; 1970:139–151.

Lowenstein A, Green WR. Retinal histology. In: Guyer DR, Yannuzzi LA, Chang S, Shields JA, Green WR, eds. *Retina-Vitreous-Macula.* Vol. 1. Philadelphia: Saunders; 1999:3–20.

Machemer R. The importance of fluid absorption, traction, intraocular currents and chorioretinal scars in the therapy of rhegmatogenous retinal detachments. *Am J Ophthalmol* 1984;98:681.

Ryan SJ, ed. *Retina.* Vol. 1, 2nd ed. St. Louis, MO: Mosby; 1994:5–123.

Schepens CL. *Retinal Detachment and Allied Diseases.* Vol. 1. Philadelphia: Saunders; 1983:23–87.

2

Preoperative Evaluation of the Retinal Detachment Patient

Stanley Chang

Thorough preoperative evaluation of the patient with retinal detachment is as important as the surgical procedure itself. After examination of the patient is completed, the surgical strategy can be planned preoperatively. Specific aspects of the management strategy to be considered are a segmental or radial buckle versus an encircling scleral buckle, the necessity for drainage of subretinal fluid, the possible need for air or gas tamponade, or the need for vitrectomy to mobilize fixed or star folds resulting from epiretinal proliferation. More recently, alternative techniques for the management of retinal detachment without permanent scleral buckling, such as a temporary parabulbar balloon or pneumatic retinopexy, may also be appropriate in selected cases. Careful study of the vitreoretinal relationships is vital to a successful result. The preoperative evaluation should include a detailed clinical history, comprehensive ophthalmic evaluation of both anterior and posterior segments of the eye, and informed consent from the patient following detailed explanation of the planned surgical procedure.

Clinical History

The duration of symptoms resulting from vitreous opacities should be determined as accurately as possible. Often patients report symptoms such as spots, lines, cobwebs, or floaters. Sometimes they will observe a mobile "veil" or "film." A history of photopsia may also be reported. Many patients are not aware of the significance of floaters or photopsia and do not seek attention until a peripheral field defect or central visual loss occurs secondary to macular detachment. Precise description of the symptoms may aid in localizing the retinal breaks. If the patient has had retinal detachment previously, the details and results of prior surgery should be obtained if possible. A previous history of ocular disease relevant to retinal detachment such as myopia, glaucoma, ocular inflammation, trauma, or cataract surgery should be documented. A family history of retinal detachment should also be noted.

There is wide variation in the ability of patients to recall their symptoms. Some patients are able to relate a very detailed history of the direction of field loss and associated symptoms, while others are unable to describe their symptoms precisely. Patients who have had a retinal detachment previously are often more alert to symptoms that may occur in the fellow eye.

Ocular Examination

The ocular examination should include a complete general eye examination as well as a detailed fundus study. The refractive error should be recorded. In eyes with a history of amblyopia, an autorefractor or retinoscopic evaluation may determine the true refractive status. The corrected visual acuity should be recorded for each eye. A confrontation visual field may determine the extent of the retinal detachment prior to funduscopic examination. An afferent pupillary defect is usually present in the affected eye. Applanation tonometry may be used to record the intraocular pressure. In most cases the intraocular pressure is lower as a result of the retinal detachment, but the presence of hypotony should raise the possibility of accompanying choroidal detachment. In patients with a history of glaucoma, the use of cycloplegic agents for preoperative pupillary dilation may cause a rise in intraocular pressure.

The lids and conjunctiva should be examined for blepharitis or conjunctivitis prior to pupillary dilation. Phenylephrine hydrochloride may constrict conjunctival blood vessels and mask an ocular infection. The presence of severe blepharitis or conjunctivitis should lead to a delay in surgery until the condition has been treated.

Limitations in ocular motility or strabismus should be measured and noted. If the patient has had previous retinal surgery and abnormalities in ocular motility are noted, the patient should be informed of the increased possibility of diplopia after the retina is reattached.

On slit-lamp examination, abnormalities in corneal clarity or size should be noted. The depth of the anterior chamber should be checked. In patients with a narrow peripheral angle, gonioscopy is indicated to avoid angle closure by pupillary dilation. Such eyes may require laser iridectomy prior to pupillary dilation and retinal detachment surgery. Any patients with a history of glaucoma or pupillary rubeosis should also undergo gonioscopy.

In patients with Marfan's syndrome or a history of ocular trauma, lens subluxation or phacodonesis may also be present. If an intraocular lens implant has been inserted, the type of implant and integrity of the posterior capsule following extracapsular cataract extraction should be noted. In aphakic patients, vitreous fibrils may be displaced anteriorly through the pupil by a bullous retinal detachment. Vitreous strands to the cataract wound should be studied. The hyaloid face may be in contact with the corneal endothelium, resulting in localized corneal edema.

In phakic patients with symptoms of posterior vitreous separation, it is helpful to examine the anterior vitreous with the slit lamp. The presence of pigment (frequently present only after vertical and horizontal eye movements) almost invariably indicates the presence of a retinal tear.

After the slit-lamp examination is completed, maximum pupillary dilation should be obtained prior to funduscopic examination. Cyclopentolate hydrochloride 1% and phenylephrine hydrochloride 2.5% (or 10% in refractory cases) can be used in combination at 20–30 minute intervals until maximum dilation occurs. In patients with iris-fixated intraocular lenses, dilation should be done more cautiously to prevent dislocation of the implant.

Examination of the Fundus

The funduscopic examination consists of three parts: (1) indirect ophthalmoscopy with scleral depression, (2) noncontact biomicroscopy of vitreoretinal relationships using an aspheric lens, and (3) contact lens examination of the retina and anterior chamber angle. The following instruments should be available:

- Indirect ophthalmoscope with small pupil attachment
- Scleral depressor
- Fundus drawing paper
- Colored pencils
- Lenses for indirect ophthalmoscopy: 14-, 20-, 25-, 28-, or 30-diopter
- 90-, 78-, or 66-diopter aspheric noncontact lenses
- Three-mirror contact lens
- Macular lens
- Panfunduscopic lens

An indirect ophthalmoscope should be chosen that is lightweight and fits comfortably, since the examination in some difficult cases may take up to 60 minutes. A small pupil attachment is helpful for poorly dilated eyes or in pseudophakic eyes with peripheral lens remnants. The room is darkened and indirect ophthalmoscopy is started when the examiner is dark adapted. The patient is placed supine on an examining chair or table. The chin is extended forward slightly. The examiner stands at the head of the patient and the fundus drawing paper is kept next to the head of the patient on the side of the examiner's writing hand or on the patient's chest. The 12 o'clock meridian of the drawing is directed toward the patient's feet and the examiner is positioned opposite to the meridian of interest and sketches exactly what is observed. By placing the drawing upside-down, one obviates the need to transpose the inverted image of the indirect ophthalmoscope. The beginning examiner should learn to hold the lens with the nondominant hand so that the writing hand can be used for drawing or scleral depression. The conventional color scheme used for fundus drawing is:

- Light blue: retinal detachment
- Dark blue: retinal veins, margins of retinal breaks
- Light red: attached retina
- Dark red: retinal arteries, preretinal or intraretinal hemorrhages
- Green: vitreous or lens opacities
- Black: chorioretinal pigmentation
- Yellow: intraretinal or subretinal exudates, subretinal bands
- Brown: choroidal detachment, nevi, or melanomas

At the beginning of the examination, the intensity of the indirect ophthalmoscope is reduced to allow the patient to adjust to the brightness of the light. Initially, a broad survey of the funduscopic findings is obtained without scleral depression. When the patient is more comfortable with the examining light, the illumination can be increased. The meridians delimiting the edges of the retinal detachment are first noted and the extent of detachment is sketched onto the fundus drawing. The fundus drawing paper (Figure 2-1) contains three concentric circles. The inner circle represents the equator of the fundus, the middle circle represents the ora serrata, and the outer band the pars plana.

Retinal breaks visible without scleral depression are localized and drawn. Following the retinal blood vessels out to the periphery allows systematic examination of the entire fundus. Scleral depression is required for examination of the peripheral retina. The patient is more comfortable when scleral depression is started temporally. The temporal periphery is more easily visualized and, as the eye softens from scleral depression, the nasal fundus can be more easily examined. Optimal visualization of the peripheral fundus is usually obtained when the examiner stands directly opposite to the meridian of interest. In patients with small pupils or peripheral lens opacities, visualization of retinal breaks may also be improved by turning the patient's head toward the examiner and asking the patient to look toward that meridian.

Specific features of the retinal detachment should be noted on the fundus drawing:

1. The relationships of retinal blood vessels and vortex veins to the location of breaks should be drawn to provide landmarks for intraoperative localization. These may be helpful during surgery if visualization decreases due to corneal edema or vitreous hemorrhage. Avulsed or bridging blood vessels over retinal tears should also be noted.
2. The height or elevation of the retinal detachment should be studied to determine whether drainage of subretinal fluid is required. More bullous areas are preferable for possible drainage sites.
3. Areas of choreoretinal pigmentation and demarcation lines should be indicated. Demarcation lines may help to localize the region of the retinal breaks.
4. Areas of peripheral lattice degeneration and areas suspicious for retinal breaks should be noted. Some of these areas will require examination under higher magnification using the contact lens.
5. When multiple breaks are present, their anteroposterior location should be accurately depicted. As a general rule, vortex veins delineated the equator and can be helpful in the precise determination of anteroposterior location. This information will be used to plan the size and extent of scleral buckling.
6. Lines of circumferential traction in the anterior retina and star or fixed folds should be indicated. By observing the mobility of the retina as the patient moves the eye, the severity of traction can be evaluated. Poor mobility indicates that the retina is stiffened by epiretinal membranes and may require vitrectomy.

The posterior pole is usually reserved for the final part of the examination with indirect ophthalmoscopy. A 14-diopter condensing lens provides higher magnification for small breaks. Macular holes, cysts, or macular pucker may be present. Posterior breaks may also be present near the edge of a staphyloma or coloboma or adjacent to larger retinal blood vessels.

When the examination is completed in the supine position, the patient is examined in the

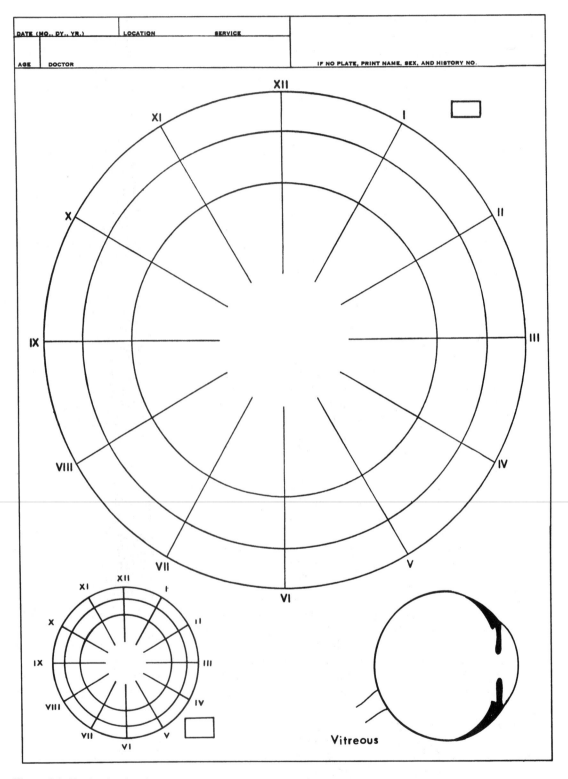

Figure 2-1. Fundus drawing document.

sitting position. This may allow folds within the retinal detachment to open, revealing previously unseen retinal breaks. The presence of shifting fluid is usually associated with exudative retinal detachments but can also be seen in patients with rhegmatogenous retinal detachments with small retinal breaks.

The patient is returned to the slit lamp and undergoes biomicroscopy using the 90-, 78-, or 66-diopter aspheric lens and three-mirror contact lens. The advantages of the aspheric lenses for funduscopic evaluation are that they allow a biomicroscopic examination without placement of a lens on the eye, and its depth of focus permits excellent visualization of vitreoretinal relationships. Areas of adhesion of the posterior hyaloid to the retina can be seen. Posterior fundus evaluation is particularly effective because of the ability to increase magnification. The beginning examiner quickly adapts to the inverted image and learns that the image moves opposite to the direction of gaze.

The three-mirror contact lens examination is an important part of fundus evaluation because it allows further magnification and refinement of the findings seen on indirect ophthalmoscopy. At higher magnification, small breaks and vitreoretinal relationships are more easily appreciated. Topical proparacaine 0.5% is instilled into the conjunctival fornix and methylcellulose solutions (1% to 2.5%) are used on the contact lens. The patient's head is placed into the slit-lamp microscope and the patient is instructed to look up while the lower lid is retracted and the lens placed onto the eye. After examination of the posterior fundus through the central lens, each of the three mirrors is used to examine the fundus. The largest mirror allows study of the post-equatorial fundus. The middle-sized mirror is used to study the pre-equatorial retinal periphery. Asking the patient to look toward the meridian of the mirror allows more posterior visualization, while looking in the meridian opposite to the mirror provides a more peripheral view. It is helpful to move the light of the slit lamp to the same side as the mirror when examining inferior quadrants of the fundus, and to direct the light from the opposite direction when studying the superior retinal quadrants. Macular lenses (contact lenses similar to the central portion of the 3-mirror contact lens) are only useful for examining the posterior pole.

The wide field of visualization of the panfunduscopic lenses can be useful in surveying the mid-peripheral fundus to the equatorial region, particularly in eyes with small pupils.

Lesions Simulating Retinal Breaks

Some peripheral retinal abnormalities may mimic retinal breaks. Small retinal hemorrhages in the region of the vitreous base may be mistaken for retinal tears because of their reddish appearance. Contact lens examination will differentiate these from true retinal breaks. Outer or inner layer retinal breaks within areas of retinoschisis may be difficult to differentiate from retinal breaks in chronic retinal detachment. Retinal tufts, or tags, may also resemble retinal breaks and should be examined carefully with scleral depression. Meridional complexes should be examined with scleral depression for small breaks at their posterior margin.

Some peripheral fundus changes may also resemble retinal detachment. Areas of white without pressure indicate vitreoretinal adhesion. If extensive, the whitish change may be mistaken for retinal detachment. These changes are more readily apparent in young patients with darkly pigmented fundi. Retinal cysts are round intraretinal collections of fluid that may be present on the inner or outer surface of the retina. Retinal cysts are frequently associated with chronic retinal detachment and disappear following surgical reattachment.

Acquired or congenital retinoschisis may be difficult to differentiate from atrophic retina present in chronic retinal detachment. A pigment demarcation line is indicative of retinal detachment, but the diagnosis may be difficult when none is present. Acquired retinoschisis is usually located in the inferotemporal quadrant and may also be present in the superotemporal quadrant; it is bilateral in 85% of cases. It often appears as a thin, convex, transparent surface and occasionally is seen with small whitish changes. Retinal breaks in either inner or outer layers will not result in retinal detachment, but when holes are present in both layers simultaneously, detachment is likely to be present.

Lincoff's Rules of Retinal Detachment

When the funduscopic examination has been completed and the location of retinal breaks found, the examiner should consider whether the configuration of the detachment is consistent with the location of the retinal breaks. Retinal detachments accumulate subretinal fluid in a predictable manner around the retinal break of origin. These observations have been extensively described and are known as Lincoff's Rules. The shape of the retinal detachment indicates the location of the break in 96% of cases.

Some concepts that may be useful in finding the break are that (1) in superonasal or temporal retinal detachments, the retinal break lies within one and one-half clock hours of the highest border 98% of the time; (2) in superior detachments that cross the midline, the primary retinal break is at 12 o'clock or within a triangle the apex of which is at the ora serrata and that intersects the equator 1 hour to either side of 12 o'clock, this is present 93% of the time; (3) in inferior detachments, the higher side indicates to which side of the 6 o'clock meridian an inferior hole lies 95% of the time; (4) when an inferior retinal detachment has a bullous configuration, the primary hole lies above the horizontal meridian.

These rules are most applicable in the absence of proliferative vitreoretinopathy since significant tractional forces can alter the distribution of subretinal fluid. If the location of the retinal breaks does not explain the retinal detachment, additional study of the retinal detachment is suggested to seek any possible missed retinal breaks.

Preoperative Informed Consent

The patient with retinal detachment is often quite apprehensive, for several reasons. The acute discovery of a retinal detachment has brought the retinal surgeon and the patient together. Usually the patient has not met the retinal surgeon until referred for evaluation of retinal detachment. Often patients have a poor understanding of the pathophysiologic processes involved in retinal detachment and the surgical procedure required for treatment. Therefore, an explanation should be provided to the patient of the events leading to the retinal detachment and the planned treatment. The overall tone should be supportive and positive since the prognosis for retinal reattachment is good. The patient should be informed of possible intraoperative as well as postoperative complications. These include complications from drainage of subretinal fluid, retinal perforation during placement of scleral sutures, choroidal detachment, macular pucker, proliferative vitreoretinopathy, or diplopia. If the macula is detached preoperatively, the prognosis for return of central vision should be indicated to the patient. Patients may not realize that it may take up to 6 months before central vision returns. Finally, the patient should be given ample opportunity to ask any questions related to the planned surgery.

Suggested Reading

Beyer NE. *The Peripheral Retina in Profile: A Stereoscopic Atlas.* Torrance, CA: Criterion Press; 1982.

Beyer NE. Peripheral retinal lesions related to rhegmatogenous retinal detachment. In: Guyer DR, Yannuzzi LA, Chang S, Shields JA, Green WR, eds. *Retina-Vitreous Macula.* Vol. 2. Philadelphia: Saunders; 1999: 1219–1247.

Brod RD, Lightman DA, Packer AJ, Saras HP. Correlation between vitreous pigment granules and retinal breaks in eyes with acute posterior vitreous detachment. *Ophthalmology* 1991;98:1366–1369.

Hilton GF, McLean EB, Brinton DA. *Retinal Detachment: Principles and Practice.* 2nd ed. San Francisco: American Academy of Ophthalmology; 1995:41–81.

Lincoff H, Gieser R. Finding the retinal hole. *Arch Ophthalmol* 1971;85:565.

Regillo CD, Benson WE. *Retinal Detachment: Diagnosis and Management.* 3rd ed. Philadelphia: Lippincott–Raven; 1998:45–99.

Schepens CLS. *Retinal Detachment and Allied Diseases.* Philadelphia: Saunders; 1983:99–232.

3

Preoperative Ophthalmic Echography and Electrophysiology

Robert E. Leonard II and Dwain G. Fuller

Ophthalmic echography and electrophysiologic studies can provide valuable aid to today's vitreoretinal surgeon in the evaluation of eyes with opaque media. Obviously, in eyes with a rhegmatogenous retinal detachment and clear media, no ancillary testing is needed for diagnosis and treatment. In contrast, an eye with a dense cataract, cyclitic membrane, hyphema, vitreous hemorrhage, or other significant opacity of the media may harbor posterior segment pathology such as a tumor or detachment that can readily be diagnosed with preoperative echography. Ophthalmic echography has emerged as a diagnostic modality that is extremely useful in the assessment of eyes with anterior or posterior segment media opacity. Electrophysiology may also be of use in the functional assessment of eyes with cloudy media to determine if there is a reasonable prospect of salvaging vision.

Echography

The development of clinical ophthalmic echography in the 1970s greatly modified and improved the management of retinal detachments and other posterior segment pathology in eyes with opaque media. The concurrent introduction of pars plana vitrectomy by Robert Machemer gave the retinal surgeon the necessary tools to approach such eyes aggressively and, in many cases, to effect dramatic visual restoration. Prior to the advent of pars plana vitrectomy, the management of retinal detachment in the presence of vitreous hemorrhage typically

included bed rest, elevation of the head, and bilateral eye patching. If the blood cleared in a timely fashion, retinal tears could be localized and scleral buckling performed. Eyes in which the vitreous hemorrhage did not clear or did not clear adequately to allow for visualization of the retinal breaks might be subjected to a so-called "blind" buckling procedure. Certainly, the advent of vitrectomy and subsequent advances in vitreoretinal surgery have allowed for earlier and more precise intervention in these cases. In an eye with media opacities that preclude visualization of the fundus, echography can quickly answer a number of questions of interest to the vitreoretinal surgeon and facilitate appropriate management.

1. Is the posterior segment anatomically normal?
2. Is the retina detached? Is there evidence of proliferative vitreoretinopathy (PVR)? Is there evidence of tractional retinal detachment?
3. Are there ultrasonographic findings that suggest a secondary retinal detachment (tumor, inflammatory condition)?
4. Are choroidal detachments (serous or hemorrhagic) present?
5. Are signs of trauma evident, such as subretinal hemorrhage, posterior rupture, intraocular foreign body, or lens luxation or disruption?
6. Is there an occult posterior tumor present, and if so, what are its characteristics?

Contact B-scan echography is the method of choice for the vitreoretinal surgeon evaluating eyes with cloudy media. Real-time dynamic B-scan echography can yield valuable information regarding the nature of a retinal detachment, allowing for the differentiation of a mobile, more acute detachment from a fixed, chronic one. Currently, three-dimensional ultrasound imaging is being evaluated for clinical application. Possible uses of three-dimensional ultrasound include volumetric analysis of tumors and more accurate assessment of complex retinal detachments.

A-scan techniques, particularly standardized A-scan echography as popularized by Karl Ossoinig, are invaluable for determining the size and characteristics of intraocular tumors. Such procedures can accurately assess the apical height of a tumor and often provide useful tissue characterization. For example, a homogenous tumor mass such as a posterior uveal melanoma would display low internal reflectivity on A-scan, whereas a vascular tumor such as a choroidal hemangioma would typically show a high internal reflectivity pattern due to its heterogeneous tissue structure.

Normal Posterior Segment

If the posterior segment is anatomically normal, the vitreous cavity will be acoustically clear or have minimal signal intensity. The retina will be attached and the choroid will not be thickened. A posterior vitreous detachment may or may not be present. Contact B-scan echography can rapidly and easily identify eyes with normal posterior segments.

Rhegmatogenous Retinal Detachment

Total retinal detachment is usually a straightforward diagnosis with echography. Highly reflective retinal leaves emanate from the optic nerve head and rejoin the globe wall anteriorly at the ora serrata. Bullous detachments are widely separated from the eye wall and have a convex configuration. In contrast, a shallow retinal detachment may remain close to the eye wall and be difficult to distinguish from other entities. A partial retinal detachment is not hard to identify if the detachment extends back to the optic nerve head. A localized detachment in the periphery, however, may sometimes be difficult to differentiate from a vitreous membrane. Detached retina is normally more reflective or echogenic (brighter on B-scan) than are vitreous membranes. Figure 3-1 shows an eye with vitreous hemorrhage and a localized retinal detachment. In this particular echogram, one can also visualize the retinal break (arrow). There is

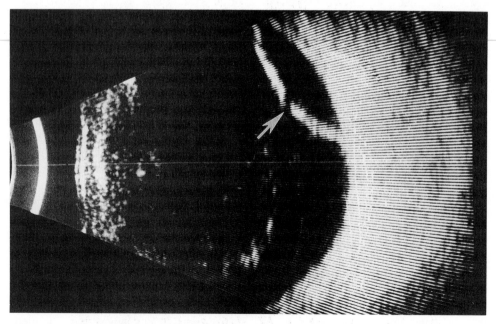

Figure 3-1. Localized rhegmatogenous retinal detachment. Arrow demonstrates retinal break. Acoustically reflective material in the vitreous cavity represents vitreous hemorrhage.

acoustically reflective material in the vitreous cavity that represents the vitreous hemorrhage. The well-differentiated membrane extending into the vitreous typifies a partial retinal detachment. The subretinal space is acoustically clear, and the tiny defect seen in the retina represents the retinal break. At surgery, a vitrectomy was performed that allowed correlation of the ultrasonographic findings with the presence of a retinal tear, a bridging retinal vessel, and a localized retinal detachment. Figure 3-2 demonstrates a retinal tear without retinal detachment. The area of vitreoretinal traction is clearly seen.

Dynamic or kinetic examination allows the examiner to determine the mobility of a detached retina. The B-scan ultrasound probe is placed on the patient's closed eyelids, allowing visualization of the detached retina. By having the patient look in various directions, characterization of the retinal detachment is possible. A nonorganized retinal detachment shows obvious, but limited after-movement at the completion of an eye duction. Vitreous membranes typically are more mobile than detached retina. In cases of significant PVR, there is little or no retinal after-movement since the retina has extensive epiretinal membrane formation and fixed folds. With advanced PVR, several different configurations may be seen. Anterior loop traction may be identified as retina is pulled up into peripheral folds with foreshortening of the posterior retina. A so-called open-funnel retinal detachment may also be seen. Figure 3-3 illustrates this type of detachment. The two retinal leaves that emanate from the optic nerve head are foreshortened and proceed to the posterior surface of the lens, indicating anterior PVR. In the most severe form of PVR, the funnel closes, with fusion of the retinal leaves, resulting in a closed-funnel retinal detachment, as shown in Figure 3-4.

The subretinal space is acoustically clear in most cases of retinal detachment; however, subretinal hemorrhage may be present in traumatic retinal detachments, nonrhegmatogenous detachments from disciform macular degeneration, or occasionally in retinal detachment from proliferative diabetic retinopathy. Figure 3-5 illustrates the appearance of subretinal hemorrhage, in this case from a disciform process. Figure 3-6 demonstrates a diabetic tractional retinal detachment with echogenic subretinal fluid and a subhyaloid hemorrhage. Subretinal particles can also be seen in some chronic retinal detachments in which mobile subretinal cholesterol crystals can develop. These particles are highly echogenic and strikingly mobile when examined using kinetic echography and provide an almost pathognomonic picture.

An organized posterior vitreous detachment (PVD), such as might be seen in an eye with

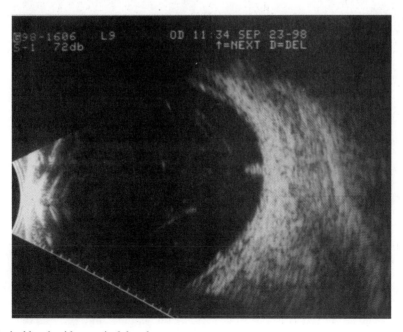

Figure 3-2. Retinal break without retinal detachment.

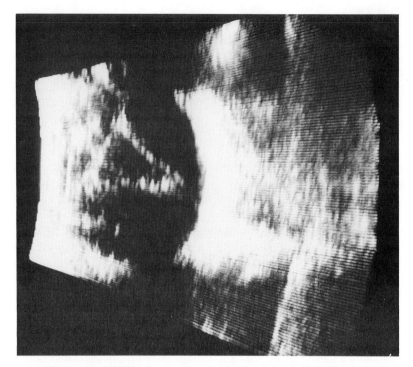

Figure 3-3. Open-funnel retinal detachment.

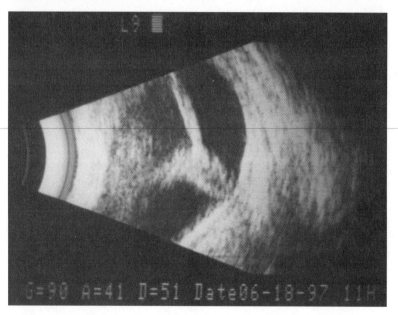

Figure 3-4. Closed-funnel retinal detachment.

previous vitreous cavity hemorrhage, can mimic ultrasonographically a total retinal detachment if the posterior vitreous face remains adherent to the optic nerve head. A PVD is usually more mobile than a total retinal detachment and often has a discontinuous border and irregular thickness on B-scan echography, but sometimes this distinction is difficult. Figure 3-7 illustrates a PVD in an eye with vitreous hemorrhage that could easily be confused with a retinal detachment. Occasionally, one can also see a stalk that attaches to the optic nerve and extends into the vitreous cavity before bifurcating into the apparent leaves of the membrane. This particular finding is characteristic of

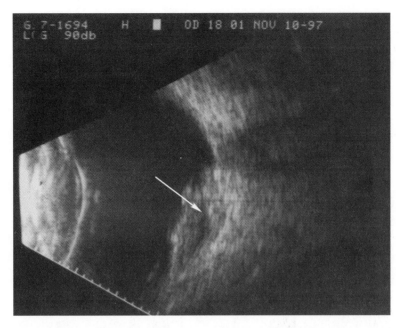

Figure 3-5. Disciform scar with subretinal hemorrhage. Subretinal blood is identified (arrow).

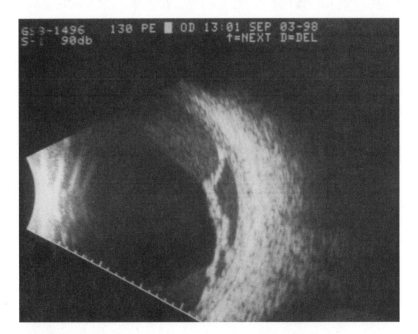

Figure 3-6. Diabetic traction retinal detachment.

PVD with a proliferative stalk at the optic nerve head, as might be seen with proliferative diabetic retinopathy. To help differentiate a PVD mimicking a retinal detachment from a true retinal detachment, bright flash electroretinography (ERG) may be performed (see the following section on electrophysiology).

Nonrhegmatogenous Retinal Detachment

It is important to remember that a retinal detachment in an eye with opaque media is not always rhegmatogenous and may be a secondary detachment. Such eyes are not candidates for vitreoretinal surgery to repair the retinal detachment, and

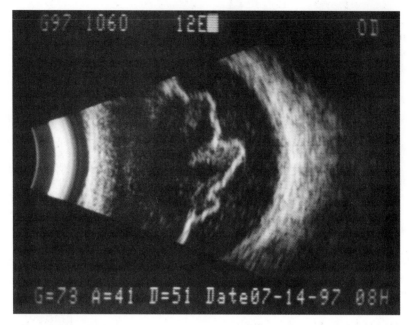

Figure 3-7. Posterior vitreous separation.

indeed, surgery on eyes containing malignant intraocular tumors such as melanoma may portend a poor systemic prognosis for the patient. A careful ultrasonographic search of the subretinal space is essential to rule out the presence of a mass lesion such as a posterior uveal melanoma, choroidal metastatic tumor, or choroidal heman-gioma. Posterior uveal melanomas may produce a vitreous hemorrhage and secondary retinal detachment that may mimic a retinal detachment unless careful echographic examination is performed. Figure 3-8 demonstrates a posterior uveal melanoma associated with a secondary retinal detachment.

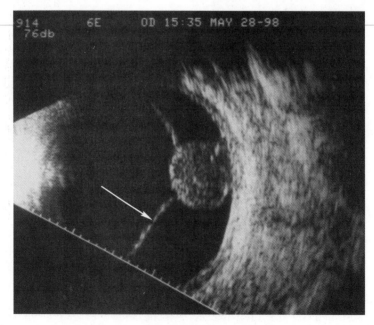

Figure 3-8. Posterior uveal melanoma. Note secondary retinal detachment (arrow).

Serous retinal detachments present in an eye with opaque media can often be confused with a rhegmatogenous retinal detachment. Shifting dependent fluid during positioning in a kinetic echographic exam can be useful in differentiating these two entities. Additionally, increased reflectivity in the subretinal fluid, a smooth convex appearance, choroidal thickening or associated choroidal detachment, and absence of a break can be helpful factors in distinguishing a serous retinal detachment from a rhegmatogenous detachment.

Choroidal Detachment

A choroidal detachment is seen echographically as a membranous structure that can be confused with a retinal detachment by the uninitiated. It is important to make this distinction, since choroidal detachment is frequently managed medically while retinal detachment often requires surgical intervention. As a general rule, a choroidal detachment is overtly convex, does not originate as far posteriorly as the optic nerve, and inserts anteriorly in front of the ora serrata. Large choroidal detachments can meet in the midvitreous cavity and give an ultrasonographic picture of "kissing" choroidals.

Choroidal detachments can be serous or hemorrhagic. Serous choroidal detachments have an acoustically clear suprachoroidal space. Figure 3-9 illustrates a serous "kissing" choroidal detachment. Note the position of the optic nerve in relationship to the choroidal detachment. Figure 3-10 demonstrates a "kissing" hemorrhagic choroidal detachment, which, in contrast to a serous choroidal detachment, has prominent echoes returning from the suprachoroidal space.

Ultrasonography can be useful in timing the drainage of suprachoroidal hemorrhage if it is required. Kinetic examination may show mobility of liquefied suprachoroidal blood in hemorrhagic choroidal detachments that are amenable to drainage. The absence of liquefied blood often indicates that a clot may be present, which makes drainage of the hemorrhagic choroidal detachment difficult.

Trauma

Echography is of extreme value in the setting of trauma, allowing for more accurate assessment of internal ocular anatomy than either conventional plain orbital radiographs or computed tomography (CT) scans. By performing a gentle exam through closed lids, many open globe injuries may be safely evaluated. Information on the status of the crystalline lens, possible intraocular foreign bodies, retinal detachment, suprachoroidal hemorrhage, and

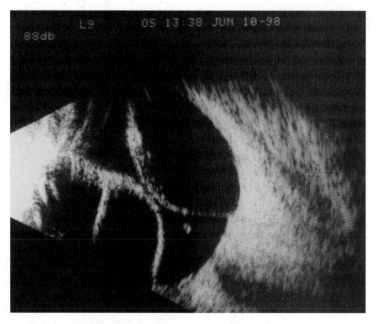

Figure 3-9. Serous appositional or so-called "kissing" choroidal detachment.

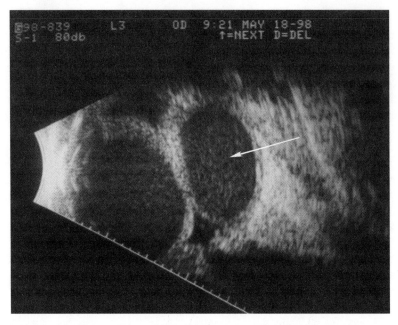

Figure 3-10. Hemorrhagic choroidal detachment. Note echogenic reflections in the suprachoroidal space (arrow).

posterior ruptures may be ascertained when no view is obtainable preoperatively.

B-scan echography can be used to identify and localize foreign bodies and determine their proximity to other ocular surfaces. Metal, glass, and plastic are highly reflective and are seen as bright acoustical point sources. Often, shadowing or loss of reflectiveness is apparent behind metallic or other echogenic intraocular foreign bodies, allowing some insight into the material involved. Plastic, nonleaded glass, and vegetable matter foreign bodies can be detected by ultrasonography, whereas plain foreign body radiographs or CT scans may miss these materials. An average foreign body diameter of 1 mm is necessary to permit easy detection and localization. While both CT- and B-scan echography are considered excellent for the detection of metallic intraocular foreign bodies, the 2-mm cuts of standard computed tomography have been reported to miss small foreign bodies that were detected by echography (Weiss, Hofeldt, and Behrens; 1997).

Foreign bodies that are near other highly reflective surfaces such as the globe wall, lens, ciliary body, or iris are more difficult to find. Figure 3-11 demonstrates such a foreign body adjacent to the globe wall (arrow). Foreign bodies that lie outside the globe may be more difficult to detect since fat is highly reflective and may mask foreign body echoes. Spherical foreign bodies such as BBs or buckshot are particularly easy to find, whether they are intraocular or extraocular. The parallel surfaces of these spherical objects cause ultrasonic reverberation within the foreign body, producing a trail of duplication echoes that extend directly behind the main foreign body echo on the ultrasound screen (Figure 3-12). A small intraocular air or gas bubble gives an identical sound pattern. Unlike the foreign body, however, the air or gas bubble can usually be mobilized during positioning of the patient's head in a kinetic examination.

Echographic identification of a hemorrhagic retinal detachment is a grave finding in an eye following trauma. Figure 3-13 illustrates such a hemorrhagic retinal detachment. Most eyes with extensive subretinal hemorrhage are lost regardless of the surgical skills employed to save the eye.

Electrophysiology

Preoperative electrophysiological studies are seldom indicated in eyes with clear media and retinal detachments. In contrast, eyes with media opacities and a possible retinal detachment or other posterior segment disease may often benefit from electrophysiologic evaluation. The two primary tests utilized are the bright-flash ERG and the flash visually evoked response (VER).

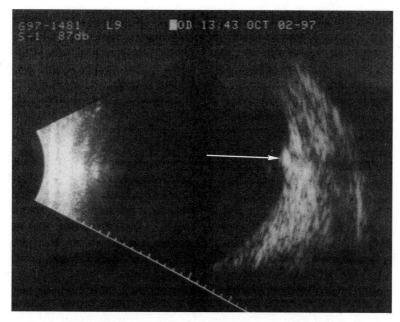

Figure 3-11. Intraocular foreign body adjacent to globe wall (arrow).

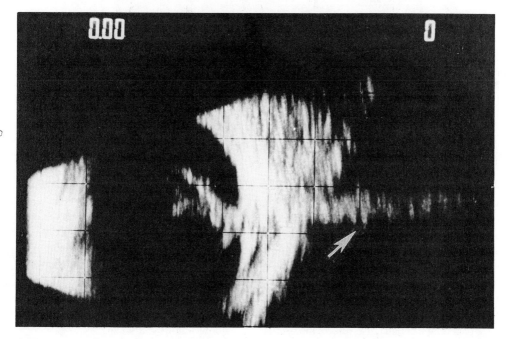

Figure 3-12. Metallic intraocular foreign body (BB). Arrow demonstrates trail of duplication echoes extending behind foreign body.

Electroretinogram

The electroretinogram (ERG) records the electrical response of the retina to photic stimulation. Two principal waves are generated; an initial negative waveform called the a-wave followed by a positive waveform, the so-called b-wave (Figure 3-14). The a-wave is derived from the outer retina (rod and cone photoreceptors), and the b-wave originates from the inner retina (Muller cells and bipolar cell layer). Also of note, but less clinically important, are c-wave and oscillatory potentials.

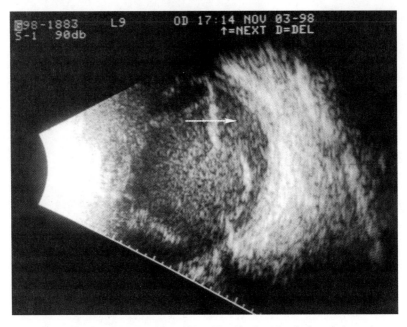

Figure 3-13. Traumatic hemorrhagic retinal detachment. Note blood in the subretinal space (arrow).

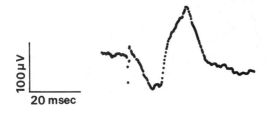

Figure 3-14. Electroretinogram (ERG).

The c-wave represents the hyperpolarization of the retinal pigment epithelium and follows the b-wave. Diffuse degenerations that effect the retinal pigment epithelium (RPE) may reduce the c-wave amplitude. Oscillatory potentials are a series of oscillating wavelets that are superimposed on the ascending b-wave. These may be useful clinically as their amplitude is decreased or absent in the presence of retinal ischemia. Therefore, the oscillatory potentials may be decreased in diabetic retinopathy, central vein occlusion, and sickle cell retinopathy.

In eyes with dense media opacities, the conventional ERG light stimulator used for eyes with clear media may not produce enough light to stimulate the retina adequately. In such cases, a camera strobe can be used to generate up to 20,000 times more light and thus stimulate the retina through major opacities. This so-called bright-flash ERG technique can be particularly useful for the vitreoretinal surgeon in evaluating the posterior segment of eyes with vitreous hemorrhage or total hyphemas. Cataracts alone do not block enough light to necessitate the use of a bright-flash stimulator.

Clinical application of the ERG is relatively straightforward if one understands a few basic principles:

1. The amplitude (height) of the a-wave corresponds with the amount of retina that is attached and functioning normally. Think of a-wave amplitude as dependent on normal nutritional support from the adjacent choriocapillaris. Total retinal detachment (serous, hemorrhagic, or exudative) or loss of perfusion of the choriocapillaris (ophthalmic artery occlusion) results in abolition of the a-wave.
2. The amplitude of the b-wave depends on normal inner retinal nutrition. Since the b-wave follows the a-wave and is initiated by it, anything that decreases the amplitude of the a-wave will of necessity decrease the amplitude of the b-wave. If the a-wave is extinguished, no b-wave can be generated. If inner retinal nutrition is compromised, but the outer retina remains intact, a

decreased b-wave amplitude will be seen in the presence of a normal a-wave amplitude.

3. No ERG is recordable in a total retinal detachment. Even minimal separation of the photoreceptors from the retinal pigment epithelium causes almost immediate loss of the ERG.

Application of the above principles allows one to predict the ERG response in various clinical conditions.

Central Retinal Artery Occlusion

The inner retina loses perfusion but the outer retina remains nourished by the choriocapillaris. Thus, the b-wave is extinguished or diminished in the presence of a normal a-wave.

Proliferative Diabetic Retinopathy

The inner retina suffers progressive loss of nutrition from small-vessel vascular compromise, causing loss of oscillatory potentials and b-wave amplitude. With worsening diabetic changes and retinal atrophy or the development of tractional retinal detachment, the a-wave also diminishes.

Central Retinal Vein Occlusion

In perfused central retinal vein occlusion (CRVO), the b-wave is mainly affected, with little effect on the a-wave. In nonperfused CRVO and in the presence of diffuse retinal edema, both the a-wave and b-wave are reduced.

Partial Retinal Detachment

The amount of reduction of a-wave amplitude corresponds roughly with the percentage of the retina detached. Therefore, a 50% retinal detachment would cause loss of one-half of the a-wave amplitude. Since the b-wave is triggered by the a-wave, approximately one-half of the b-wave amplitude would be lost.

Bright-flash ERG can be particularly helpful in an eye with no fundus view and an apparent total retinal detachment seen by ultrasonography. A densely organized PVD that remains attached at the optic nerve head can simulate a total retinal detachment, as mentioned earlier. In such cases, the presence of a good-bright flash ERG response excludes the possibility of a total retinal detachment and establishes the diagnosis.

Visually Evoked Potential

The visually evoked potential (VEP), also known as the visually evoked cortical potential (VECP), or visually evoked response (VER), represents the summated electrical signal generated at the visual cortex in response to visual stimulation of the retina. The VEP is smaller and buried within the electroencephalogram (EEG). A normal VEP response requires not only a functional macula but also an intact visual pathway from the macula to the visual cortex. Since VEP responses are so small in amplitude, it is necessary to use a signal-averaging computer to summate responses.

Unlike the ERG, which assesses overall retinal function, the VEP specifically evaluates the integrity of the central 6–12 degrees of visual field. Thus, the VEP provides information in eyes with opaque media that is available by no other means of testing. An eye with cloudy media and count fingers visual potential due to a macular scar can have a perfectly normal ERG response. In contrast, such an eye would have a severely reduced or absent VEP response. Likewise, an eye with opaque media and grossly compromised optic nerve function would have a normal ERG, but an obviously abnormal VEP.

The light stimulus for eliciting a VEP may be a pattern such as a checkerboard or a simple flash stimulator. In eyes with opaque media, only a flash stimulator can be used. Fuller and Hutton (1982) have described a VEP technique for assessing macular and optic nerve function in eyes with opaque media by using 10, 20, and 30 flashes per second. This technique generates "steady state" VEP sinusoidal waveforms that can be evaluated simply by measuring amplitudes only (Figure 3-15). With this method, it is possible for the vitreoretinal surgeon to assess postoperative visual potential in eyes with nonvisualized posterior segments. In eyes with opaque media following severe trauma, the VEP is the single best predictor of postoperative visual

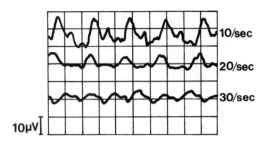

Figure 3-15. Bright-flash VEP.

recovery. It must be remembered, however, that an eye with a macular detachment will have a poor or nonrecordable VEP despite the potential for the return of useful vision following successful surgical repair.

Conclusion

Access to ultrasonography is essential for the vitreoretinal surgeon and has become an integral part of the preoperative evaluation of any eye with opaque media. Electrophysiology, although of less practical value than ultrasonography, gives the vitreoretinal surgeon an added dimension in the preoperative evaluation of eyes with opaque media and can be a distinct aid in the prediction of postoperative visual function in traumatized eyes with cloudy media.

Suggested Reading

Coleman DJ, Jack RL. B-scan ultrasonography in the diagnosis and management of retinal detachments. *Arch Ophthalmol* 1973;90:29.

Coleman DJ, Lizzi FL, Jack RL. *Ultrasonography of the Eye and Orbit.* Philadelphia: Lea & Febiger; 1977.

Cusumano A, Coleman DJ, Silverman RH, et al. Three-dimensional ultrasound imaging-clinical applications. *Ophthalmol* 1998;105:300–306.

Fuller, DG. Assessment of visual potential in eyes with densely opaque media. *Ophthalmology Clinics of North America* Sept. 1989;2(3).

Fuller DG, Hutton WL. *Presurgical Evaluation of Eyes with Opaque Media.* Orlando, FL: Grune & Stratton; 1982.

Fuller DG, Hutton WL. Prediction of postoperative vision in eyes with severe trauma. *Retina* 1990;10:S20–S34.

Fuller DG, Knighton RW, Machemer R. Bright-flash electroretinography for evaluation of eyes with opaque vitreous. *Am J Ophthalmol* 1975;80:214.

Fuller DG, Laqua H, Machemer R. Ultrasonographic diagnosis of massive periretinal proliferation in eyes with opaque media (triangular retinal detachment). *Am J Ophthalmol* 1977;83:460.

Hirose T, Miyake Y, Hara A. Evaluation of severe ocular trauma: electroretinogram and visual evoked response. In: Freeman HM, ed. *Ocular Trauma.* East Norwalk, CT: Appleton-Century-Crofts; 1979:31.

Huber CH. Amplitude versus frequency characteristics of visually evoked cortical potentials to sine wave modulated light in disease of the optic nerve. In: Lawwill T, ed. *ERG, VER, and Psychophysics: 14th I.S.C.E.R.G. Symposium.* Louisville, KY: Junk Publishers; 1977.

Hutton WL, Fuller DG. Factors influencing final visual results in severely injured eyes. *Am J Ophthalmol* 1984;97:715.

Jack RL, Hutton WL, Machemer R. Ultrasonography and vitrectomy. *Am J Ophthalmol* 1974;78:265.

Kelley LM, Walker JP, Schepens CL, et al. Ultrasound-guided cryotherapy for retinal tears in patients with vitreous hemorrhage. *Ophthalmic Surg Lasers* 1997;28:565–569.

Sokol S. Visually evoked potentials: theory, techniques and clinical applications. *Surv Ophthalmol* 1976;21:18.

Srebo R, Wright WW. Visually evoked potentials to pseudo-random binary sequence stimulation. Preliminary clinical trials. *Arch Ophthalmol* 1980;98:296.

Weinstein GW. Clinical aspects of the visual evoked potential. *Ophthalmic Surg* 1978;9:56.

Weiss MJ, Hofeldt AJ, Behrens M, et al. Ocular siderosis: diagnosis and management. *Retina* 1997;17:105–108.

4

Laser Photocoagulation
and Cryopexy of Retinal Breaks

David W. Parke II

Retinal breaks, whether atrophic retinal holes, oper-culated retinal holes, retinal dialyses, or retinal tears with a flap under vitreous traction (horseshoe tears), may be associated with retinal detachments. Under certain circumstances, the ophthalmologist may wish to treat these breaks prophylactically to reduce the chances of the development of a clinical retinal detachment.

There are five major steps in this process.

1. Detection of the retinal break(s)
2. Making a treatment decision
3. Selection of treatment modality
4. Treatment of the retinal break(s)
5. Follow-up of treatment

Detection of Retinal Break(s)

The vast majority of retinal breaks are asymptomatic. They are discovered on routine examination of the peripheral retina by indirect ophthalmoscopy or by slit lamp biomicroscopic examination either using a contact lens with angled mirrors (such as a Goldmann 3-mirror lens) or a noncontact lens (such as a 78- or 90-diopter lens). Although the prevalence of retinal breaks has been reported to lie between 4% and 18%, it is generally accepted that the prevalence of asymptomatic retinal breaks in the general population is approximately 6%.[1] Certain patients, although asymptomatic, should be considered at higher risk for retinal breaks and should be exam-ined with a higher index of suspicion. This includes patients with a history of retinal detachment in the fellow eye; a strong family history of retinal detach-ment; high myopia; disorders associated with vitre-oretinal traction and retinal detachment such as lattice degeneration and Stickler's syndrome; aphakia; or pseudophakia with anterior segment vit-reous adhesions or incarceration.

Symptomatic retinal breaks are much less com-mon than asymptomatic ones. They are generally associated with spontaneous detachment (separa-tion) of the posterior vitreous. This detachment and subsequent anterior migration of the posterior bor-der of the vitreous may induce traction in an area of vitreoretinal adhesion, resulting in tearing of the retina. Such tears become symptomatic when they are accompanied by light flashes (photopsia) or the sudden appearance of new floaters. These floaters (which may represent pigmented cells, red blood cells, or posterior vitreous condensation) are described by the patient as "spots," or (if they are more numerous) "lines" or "clouds." A posterior vitreous condensation may also be described as a "cobweb" or a "fishnet." The photopsia may occur only once or may occur repeatedly over a period of days or weeks. Although these photopsia are gener-ally noticed in the temporal visual field, this has no value for localizing the retinal break.

Every patient with the sudden onset of photop-sia and/or floaters does not necessarily have a reti-nal break. However, all such patients (unless they are known to have an unrelated disease causing these symptoms) deserve a careful examination to determine if a break is present. Although vitreous hemorrhage may accompany a posterior vitreous detachment unassociated with a retinal break, the finding of red blood cells or frank vitreous hemorrhage should particularly alert the examiner to the possibility of a retinal break. Finding pigment cells in the vitreous is also highly associated with the possibility of a coexisting retinal break.

Indirect ophthalmoscopy with scleral indentation (also known as scleral depression) remains the most valuable method of finding retinal breaks. Although many breaks can be discovered without the use of scleral indentation, tiny breaks, anteriorly located breaks, atrophic breaks, and breaks in highly myopic or lightly pigmented eyes may be easily overlooked if scleral indentation is not performed. Scleral indentation also permits more accurate determination of the presence and amount of subretinal fluid surrounding a break.

Most comprehensive ophthalmologists do not use biomicroscopic examination of the peripheral retina on a routine basis. However, biomicroscopic examination of the peripheral retina using a contact or noncontact lens can be valuable when a break is suspected but not clearly visualized by indirect ophthalmoscopy with scleral depression. (A noncontact lens is preferred by many retina subspecialists over a contact lens, as it avoids the use of contact lubricants that can make subsequent indirect ophthalmoscopy difficult.)

If a small, difficult to visualize retinal break is discovered, the examiner should take careful note of the location of the break in relation to other more easily visualized fundus landmarks such as chorioretinal scars, retinal vessels, vortex veins and ampullae, and others. This will greatly facilitate localizing the break during later treatment.

Decisions Regarding Treatment: Is Treatment Necessary?

If a retinal break is discovered on indirect ophthalmoscopy or biomicroscopic examination, the patient must be informed of the findings, their significance, and the management options. Only then can an appropriate management decision be reached. As will be noted below, a decision to treat or not to treat is sometimes quite obvious to the ophthalmologist

and is supported by statistically valid data. In most situations, however, data do not currently exist to clearly direct a management decision. Available incomplete data and the risks and benefits of therapeutic options must be presented to the patient. In the hands of an experienced surgeon, the treatment of retinal breaks should be associated with a very, very low incidence of complications. However, this infrequency of complications should not be translated into a rationale to treat all breaks. Treatment of most asymptomatic retinal breaks is not substantiated by available prospective data. Therefore, while treatment may carry a very low frequency of complications, it can be associated with discomfort and substantial cost, and may be ultimately unnecessary.

If most retinal breaks led to retinal detachment, the relative incidence of breaks would be similar to that of retinal detachment. The incidence of clinical retinal detachment (0.01–0.02%) is much lower than that for the discovery of retinal breaks. Byer, in a long-term prospective follow-up of 235 eyes with asymptomatic retinal breaks (including 46 eyes with traction retinal tears), detected no subsequent clinical retinal detachment from the nontreated tears.[2]

Even the treatment of lesions in certain groups of "high-risk" eyes has not been statistically validated. A large prospective trial treating vitreoretinal pathology in fellow eyes of retinal detachment patients in Israel concluded that treatment conferred no significant benefit.[3] Yet another study observed that it is not preexisting pathology that causes subsequent retinal detachments, but new breaks in retina previously felt to be normal.[4]

How does the ophthalmologist determine which breaks require treatment? Certain criteria—some "hard" and some "soft"—can assist in making this clinical judgment.

Symptoms

The presence or absence of associated symptoms (photopsia and/or new floaters within several weeks of examination) is the most important determinant of risk. In one series, symptomatic breaks were associated with subsequent clinical retinal detachment formation in about 30% of cases.[5] Therefore, any break associated with fresh symptoms of photopsia and/or floaters should be strongly considered for treatment.

Tear versus Operculated Retinal Break versus Atrophic Retinal Break

The risk associated with the various types of asymptomatic breaks has not been well quantified. In his series, Merin et al. discovered that 19% of fellow eyes had retinal breaks, 15% of which later developed retinal detachments.[6] Of those detachments, 71% came from flap (or "horseshoe") tears and only 19% of the breaks were tears.

Tractional retinal tears, as noted above, are more frequently associated with symptoms and are therefore of more clinical significance. However, it is not uncommon to find tractional tears that, by virtue of their appearance and associated pigment epithelial reaction, have clearly been present for months if not years. Therefore, asymptomatic tractional tears themselves do not necessarily confer a poor prognosis. As noted above, Byer evaluated 50 tractional tears for up to 18 years without treatment and without any subsequent retinal detachment. Although the strongest data favoring treatment of horseshoe tears are for symptomatic tears, some ophthalmologists believe that all tractional tears should be treated. Others believe that the treatment decision should be made on the basis of associated factors such as symptoms, myopia, family history, status of the fellow eye, and lenticular status (phakia, aphakia, pseudophakia, and impending pseudophakia).

Atrophic retinal holes with or without associated lattice degeneration constitute a very common type of retinal break. They are very rarely symptomatic. Furthermore, it is questionable whether they are responsible for symptoms even when associated with them. Pathophysiologically, they are not associated with vitreous traction but with progressive retinal atrophic changes. As such, they are very rarely associated with retinal detachments and therefore rarely require treatment.

Operculated retinal breaks are felt to generally be low risk lesions as well. As the flap of the tear pulls free under vitreous traction creating the operculum, traction on the break is usually relieved. Occasionally, however, vitreous traction will remain to the retina surrounding the hole. If such traction is detected or strongly suspected, such lesions may be considered for treatment.

Phakia/Aphakia/Pseudophakia

The incidence of retinal detachment in aphakic eyes is clearly higher than in phakic eyes. Several small series have suggested that the incidence of retinal detachment in aphakic eyes with known retinal breaks is substantially higher than in a similar phakic group. Population-based studies have indicated that the risk of retinal detachment is 6 to 7 times higher following modern cataract surgery than in phakic control groups.[7]

The risk of various types of retinal breaks in the pseudophakic eye has not been clearly elucidated. There is, for example, no clear assessment of the risk of asymptomatic retinal breaks to the pseudophakic eye. It is clear, however, that the risk of retinal detachment is much higher in the eye with an open posterior capsule than when the capsule is intact.[8] This is probably related to factors including acceleration of the posterior vitreous detachment, changes in the chemical constitution of the vitreous and/or anterior movement of the anterior vitreous. While all symptomatic breaks should probably be treated and all asymptomatic atrophic holes should probably not be treated, lesions of intermediate risk (such as an asymptomatic flap tear) are deemed by many (in the absence of good data) to be higher risk in pseudophakic than in phakic eyes.

Good data do not exist to help guide management decisions in phakic eyes with lesions of intermediate risk that will shortly undergo cataract surgery or in pseudophakic eyes scheduled for YAG capsulotomy. Treatment in such cases should be individualized taking into account patient demographics, associated risk factors, and the characteristics of the lesion in question.

Myopia

Myopia has been considered an important factor by some in electing to treat asymptomatic retinal breaks. Studies published by the Eye Disease Case-Control Study Group and by Burton have demonstrated that myopia from 1 to 3 diopters is associated with a fourfold increase in retinal detachment risk and that higher myopia is associated with a ten times increased risk.[9,10] However, patients with highly myopic eyes also have an increased prevalence of asymptomatic retinal breaks over the general population. Therefore, asymptomatic retinal breaks in myopia may not confer a statistically worse prognosis than in emmetropia. Neumann and Hymas reported in 1972 that only one clinical retinal detachment occurred in a group of 75 myopic eyes with retinal breaks evaluated for 2 years without treatment.[11] The one break that did progress to a clinical detachment was a 90-degree tractional tear. Byer noted a statistical association between high myopia and subclinical retinal detachments but not with clinical retinal detachments.[2] The high risk of retinal detachment following cataract extraction in high myopia (12–30%) has led some ophthalmologists to recommend treatment of retinal breaks in aphakic or pseudophakic highly myopic eyes as well as in highly myopic phakic eyes prior to cataract surgery.

Fellow Eyes

A history of retinal detachment in one eye clearly confers a higher than normal risk for retinal detachment in the fellow eye. Several studies have indicated that prophylactic treatment of retinal tears in the fellow eye appears to lower the subsequent risk for retinal detachment.[4] While this has not been validated by a large prospective study, most ophthalmologists use this information as a basis for treating tears in fellow eyes of patients with prior retinal detachments, particularly if cataract surgery or YAG capsulotomy is scheduled.

Associated Subretinal Fluid

It is not uncommon to find subretinal fluid associated with retinal breaks, either symptomatic or asymptomatic. Strictly speaking, this constitutes a retinal detachment. However, such detachments are considered subclinical or limited if the fluid extends less than two disc diameters posterior to the equator. Therefore, even a circumferentially extensive area of subretinal fluid that remains anterior to the equator is still subclinical. Some subclinical retinal detachments are clearly chronic (based on the associated demarcation lines and changes in the underlying retinal pigment epithelium). It is not rare to find multiple subclinical retinal detachments associated with atrophic holes and lattice degeneration.

There are no data to suggest that these subclinical detachments are associated with a higher incidence of clinical retinal detachment. The association of substantial (but subclinical) subretinal fluid with tractional tears is considered by most to be an indication for treatment.

Other Factors

A number of other factors are occasionally invoked in making a decision regarding treatment. Large tears and superior tears are thought by some to carry a worse prognosis. There is no statistical information to validate this clinical impression.

Lattice degeneration by itself (separated from other previously mentioned factors) does not appear statistically to confer an additional risk.[12] Some ophthalmologists believe that asymptomatic retinal tears at the edge of patches of lattice degeneration warrant treatment because of the associated strong vitreoretinal adhesions.

The institution of miotic therapy in patients with high myopia or aphakia has been associated with retinal detachment. Therefore some ophthalmologists recommend prophylactic treatment of tears in patients with these findings prior to beginning miotic therapy.

Conditions such as Ehlers-Danlos syndrome and Stickler's syndrome are associated with a higher risk of retinal detachment. It is not clear whether this risk is due to the associated myopia or to the vitreoretinal pathology inherent in these syndromes. Tractional tears in patients with these conditions are generally considered to warrant therapy, regardless of symptoms.

It has also been suggested that treatment decisions be based in large measure on the relationship of the tear to the vitreous base.[13] Tears are thus categorized as oral if they occur at the ora serrata, intrabasal if they occur within the vitreous base, juxtabasal if they occur at the posterior border of the vitreous base, and extrabasal if they are located posterior to the vitreous base. Sigelman has suggested criteria for treatment based in large part on this classification. He argues that juxtabasal tears carry the highest risk of retinal detachment of all postora tears, and intrabasal tears carrying the lowest risk.

Of all the factors noted above, the presence of associated symptoms is the most compelling argument for the treatment of retinal tears. All other factors are supported by less compelling scientific data. Treatment decisions depend in part on the association of various factors and the clinical experience and predisposition of the physician involved. This is not to say that only symptomatic breaks should be treated, but for these the clearest statistical rationale for treatment exists. Certainly most ophthalmologists would recommend treating a large retinal tear in a highly myopic aphakic or pseudophakic eye, even one without symptoms. On the other hand, few ophthalmologists would recommend treatment of an asymptomatic atrophic retinal hole in a phakic patient as there exists no data to support this action.

Selection of Treatment Modality

There are two basic options for the treatment of peripheral retinal breaks with or without an associated subclinical retinal detachment: cryopexy and laser photocoagulation. Only rarely would other more invasive treatments (cryopexy or laser photocoagulation in combination with either intravitreal gas injection, use of an extrascleral balloon, scleral buckling, or primary vitrectomy) be considered.

These other modalities have essentially no place in the management of simple retinal breaks. They may be used occasionally if there is associated extensive subretinal fluid, profound vitreoretinal traction, or significant vitreous hemorrhage.

Cryopexy

Cryopexy involves the use of a nitrous oxide or carbon dioxide probe applied to the scleral or conjunctival surface, which causes transscleral freezing with an iceball extending to the pigment epithelium and usually the retina. The inflammatory reaction mediated by the freezing (and thawing) creates a choroidal/retinal pigment epithelial/retinal adhesion. Studies have shown that tight desmosomal connections have formed between the retina and retinal pigment epithelium by 8–12 days following application.[14] This follows cellular disruption owing to destruction of cell membranes. The amount of necrosis appears to be correlated with the size and extent of the freeze.

Within 2 weeks of cryopexy, adjacent retinal pigment epithelial (RPE) cells slide in to replace the cells disrupted by freezing. Desmosomal connections form between the RPE cells and the overlying Müllers cells. Over subsequent weeks and months the scar undergoes remodeling, with interdigitation between the RPE and adjacent Müllers cell plasma membranes. The maximum strength of the cryoadhesion appears to occur between 1 and 2 weeks following treatment.

Advantages

Cryopexy has several advantages as a treatment modality. It can be performed in conjunction with topical, subconjunctival, or retrobulbar anesthesia. Treatment of most retinal breaks requires very few applications and is generally easy to perform without a conjunctival incision for any tear from the equator to the ora serrata. It is generally performed as an outpatient procedure in the office. It is particularly useful in cases where visibility is compromised by vitreous hemorrhage, a pseudophakos edge, lens opacities, or an opacified peripheral posterior capsule.

Disadvantages

Cryopexy also has several disadvantages. It is difficult to treat more posterior breaks in most eyes unless the probe is placed subconjunctivally. It is associated with more inflammation than is laser photocoagulation and with more postoperative lid swelling and conjunctival chemosis. If topical anesthesia alone is used, it is frequently associated with moderate to severe discomfort. For this reason, many surgeons will at least supplement topical anesthesia with subconjunctival anesthesia.

Complications

Complications of treatment are few. A recent retrospective study by Roseman and colleagues of 241 eyes with retinal breaks and subclinical detachments treated by transconjunctival cryopexy revealed anatomic retinal attachment in 95% of the cases.[15] Epiretinal membrane formation (premacular fibrosis) sufficient to cause visual symptoms occurred in some eyes following cryopexy. The overall incidence is probably between 1% and 4%.

The role of cryopexy in epiretinal membrane formation is unclear. The RPE cells responsible in part for the membrane can migrate through the retinal break without cryopexy or at the time of cryopexy. It is important to note that clinically and experimentally cryopexy does result in liberation of viable pigment epithelial cells into the vitreous cavity.[16]

The progression of a very small number of retinal breaks (or retinal breaks associated with subclinical detachments) to clinical detachments following cryopexy may occasionally be related to the cryopexy itself. Extensive cryopexy can be associated with intraocular inflammation and fluid exudation (of choroidal origin) into the subretinal space. These factors, alone or in combination, may result rarely in retinal detachment. Some retina surgeons also believe that extensive cryopexy may be associated with sufficient dispersion of retinal pigment epithelial cells and inflammation as to stimulate the formation of proliferative vitreoretinopathy. This has not been proven.

Laser Photocoagulation

Laser photocoagulation is also a very efficacious mode of therapy for retinal breaks with or without surrounding subclinical retinal detachment. The laser energy results in damage to the RPE (where most of the laser energy is actually absorbed), the outer retina, and the choriocapillaris. This results in a retinal–RPE bond similar ultrastructurally to that from cryopexy. (The individual lesions are, of course, smaller.) Several studies have also suggested that the mechanical adhesion formed by photocoagulation appears somewhat earlier following laser photocoagulation than following cryopexy with at least some adhesion present immediately following the laser treatment.

Advantages

Laser photocoagulation has a number of practical advantages. Like cryopexy, it can be performed in association with topical, subconjunctival, or rarely retrobulbar anesthesia. With clear media and good pupillary dilation, it can be used to treat lesions from the ora serrata to the posterior pole. It is particularly useful for the treatment of more posterior breaks. It appears to be associated with less vitre-

ous inflammation and exudation. Laser photocoagulation is also experimentally associated with less liberation of viable RPE cells into the vitreous cavity than is cryopexy. It is not clear whether this is due to the biomechanics of the laser scar itself or to the more precise (and generally less extensive) treatment that the fine control of laser photocoagulation permits.

There are no large studies comparing the clinical results of laser photocoagulation and cryopexy for retinal breaks. However, it appears that laser photocoagulation is at least as efficacious as cryopexy. There are reasons to suspect that it might be associated with less epiretinal membrane formation than cryopexy (although these data are not available).

Disadvantages

Like cryopexy, laser photocoagulation of the peripheral retina can also be somewhat painful. Because more precise control of spot location is necessary, it may be more difficult to perform in the photosensitive patient who cannot maintain relatively good control of fixation. It may also be impossible to perform far peripheral treatment in the presence of poor pupillary dilation, peripheral cortical or (in the pseudophakic patient) of peripheral capsular opacification or dispersion of laser energy by the edge of a pseudophakos.

Which Laser Wavelength Should Be Used?

The longer exposure times, deeper burns, and increased discomfort associated with longer wavelength (particularly red) laser treatment probably constitute a minor argument in favor of green wavelengths for transpupillary laser. Diode lasers have also been used in a transconjunctival fashion for treatment of peripheral breaks, but are not widely employed for office-based treatment.

Cryopexy versus Laser Photocoagulation

In summary, both treatment modalities appear to be highly efficacious and associated with a very low incidence of side effects and complications. Many retinal breaks can be treated with equal facility with either form of therapy. In general, cryopexy is most useful for anterior breaks and eyes with media opacities. In each of these cases, visualization may be inadequate for slit lamp laser photocoagulation. (Indirect ophthalmoscope-delivered laser can be performed in many such cases.) Cryopexy or indirect ophthalmoscope-delivered laser photocoagulation are also the options of choice in small children and others who will not cooperate for laser photocoagulation (and must be sedated).

Laser photocoagulation is definitely easier than cryopexy in more posterior breaks. It is also generally easy to perform regardless of break location in adults with good dilation and no peripheral lens opacities. Even the most anterior of breaks can frequently be treated with an indirect delivery system and scleral indentation. Laser also possesses theoretical advantages in eyes with large breaks or those requiring extensive treatment, since it induces less inflammation and less RPE cell dispersion. It is also frequently a more comfortable procedure for the patient, and is associated with no postoperative lid or conjunctival swelling. Most importantly, however, laser is associated with less exudation of fluid than cryo and it experimentally appears to form a biomechanical adhesion between retina and RPE more rapidly than does cryopexy.

Treatment Technique

Cryopexy

The patient should be placed in the supine position, either in an examining chair or on an examining or operating table. Topical, subconjunctival, or retrobulbar anesthesia may be used. In general most treatment can be performed comfortably with the use of subconjunctival lidocaine (Xylocaine) 1% or 2%. This can be administered using a 30-gauge needle and tuberculin syringe following topical anesthesia with proparacaine 0.5% and lidocaine 2% on a cotton-tipped applicator applied to the injection site. If retrobulbar anesthesia is used, the resulting akinesia may require that a muscle hook or scleral depressor be used to rotate the eye into a position where the retinal break can be visualized and the cryoprobe easily positioned.

A nitrous oxide or carbon dioxide cryoprobe may be used. The probe should be primed so that the probe tip temperature of –50°C to –80°C is achieved within several seconds. The probe should be placed on the conjunctiva and the patient asked to look in a direction that allows easy indentation of the borders of the retinal break or subretinal fluid by the tip of the cryoprobe (Figure 4-1A). Care should be taken to ensure that the indentation visible ophthalmoscopically is caused by the probe tip and not by the probe shaft. If the shaft is indenting the sclera, either no visible freeze will occur (the tip is not applied against the globe) or the freeze will be much more posterior than intended (Figure 4-1B).

The area to be treated should then be frozen with the cryoprobe. In general, the ophthalmologist

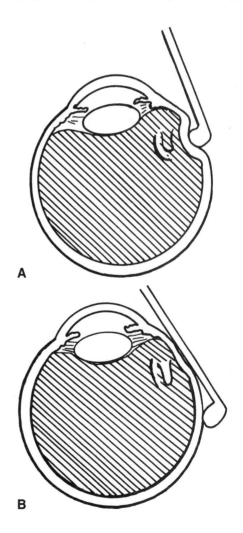

A

B

Figure 4-1. A, Scleral indentation at the retinal break by the tip of the cryoprobe. **B,** "False" scleral indentation at the retinal break by the cryoprobe shaft.

should aim for a 1–2-mm diameter area of retinal whitening. This can usually be achieved by releasing the foot-pedal the instant retinal whitening is first observed. Do not overfreeze. A single retinal freeze should not be allowed to enlarge to cover a large retinal break. This results in extreme necrosis of the center of the cryo reaction, encourages pigment epithelial cell liberation, and increases the inflammatory reaction. It is preferable to use multiple, overlapping small cryo marks rather than one, single, large cryo mark (Figure 4-2).

After each freeze has been stopped, do not move the cryoprobe immediately but wait until there has been thawing of the probe from the conjunctiva. This can be facilitated by irrigating the tip of the cryoprobe with balanced salt solution. Premature movement of the cryoprobe can result in subconjunctival, episcleral, or, rarely, choroidal hemorrhaging. After the iceball has vanished ophthalmoscopically, there may be no visible residual of the freeze. (Occasionally a faint gray color will persist.) Therefore, the ophthalmologist should carefully note the location of each zone of retinal whitening to allow proper overlapping of cryo marks without retreatment or skipped areas of nontreatment.

If no iceball is visible ophthalmoscopically after a reasonable period of freezing (4–6 seconds depending on the cryo unit), check (1) to make sure the cryoprobe tip is directly applied against the sclera (not on the lid, angled improperly, or over a rectus muscle; a longer freeze may be necessary in this last case) and (2) to ensure proper machine function (gas pressure, probe function).

Which specific area should be treated? If no subretinal fluid is present, treatment should be directed to the borders of the retinal break. There is no purpose in treating the bare RPE in the middle of the retinal break. (There is no overlying retina in this area to create an adhesive bond.) The surgeon should attempt to leave a 1-disc-diameter margin of cryo reaction around all edges of the retinal break. If the break is under significant traction, a wider zone of treatment should be placed anteriorly in case there is further enlargement of the break anteriorly from traction on the flap. If a sufficient margin cannot be created between the break and the ora serrata, treatment should be extended anteriorly to the ora serrata on each side of the break.

If there is subretinal fluid, treatment should be directed at the borders of the subretinal fluid rather than at the borders of the retinal break (Figure 4-3). Cryopexy will not generally cause resolution of the subretinal fluid. Therefore, treatment of borders of the break will result in no adhesion because of the physical separation of the RPE and retina caused by the subretinal fluid. Treatment must therefore be directed at the border between attached and detached retina. Again, if fluid extends anteriorly to the ora serrata, treatment must be extended to the ora serrata.

Following cryopexy, the patient should be instructed to use cold compresses or ice packs to reduce lid swelling. If there has been extensive treatment, the surgeon may wish to use topical corticosteroids for 3–5 days to decrease conjunctival inflammation.

Laser Photocoagulation

Most patients can be treated comfortably under topical anesthesia. In some patients, retrobulbar anes-

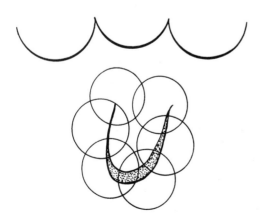

Figure 4-2. Proper application of the multiple cryo spots.

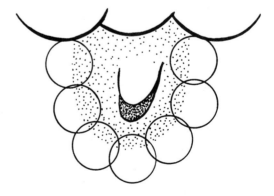

Figure 4-3. Proper application of cryo spots to surround subretinal fluid and link with the ora serrata.

thesia may be necessary. Using a slit lamp delivery system, once the retinal break has been located using a contact lens, a test burn should be placed in nearby attached retina. A 200-mm or, preferably, a 500-mm spot size should be utilized. A duration of 0.1 or 0.2 seconds can be used. Generally, power settings in the range of 100–300 mW with a green wavelength laser will be required for the desired gray-white retina/RPE burn for a 200-mm spot size; power settings of 200–500 mW are typically used for a 500-mm spot size. It is safest to start with lower power settings and work upward. If an indirect ophthalmoscope delivery system is utilized, similar spot durations should be employed with power settings to achieve the same visible gray-white endpoint.

If no subretinal fluid is present, the borders of the retinal break should be surrounded by a double or triple row of confluent laser photocoagulation (Figure 4-4). If the break is under traction, a more generous treatment margin should be placed anteriorly to provide a good margin of treatment in the event of further anterior tearing of the retina from traction on the flap. If the break is close to the ora serrata, treatment should be extended anteriorly to the ora serrata.

If subretinal fluid is present, treatment should again be directed at the attached retina just beyond the border of attached and detached retina. There is no purpose in attempting to treat detached retina.

Occasionally, laser photocoagulation will be difficult to achieve in the very far peripheral retina just posterior to the ora serrata. This is particularly true in cases of cataract, poor pupillary dilation, or optical aberration from a posterior chamber intraocular

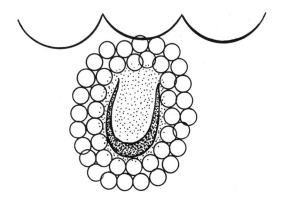

Figure 4-4. Proper application of laser burns around a retinal break.

lens or peripheral posterior capsule opacification. In these situations, it may be necessary to place one or several cryo marks to link the most anterior aspect of the laser photocoagulation with the ora serrata or to use the indirect ophthalmoscope-delivered laser.

Following laser photocoagulation there is generally no need for topical medication.

Follow-Up Care

In general, the patient should be instructed to return for a follow-up evaluation about one week following treatment. There are no data to suggest that restriction of activity plays any role in efficacy of treatment or in later complications. In general a satisfactory ophthalmoscopic appearance at 1 week following treatment will be associated with a satisfactory eventual outcome, although patients should generally be reevaluated again within 3 to 6 weeks. At these examinations care should be taken to assure that subretinal fluid has not extended through the prior treatment. If this has occurred, the patient should generally be retreated.

It is important to counsel patients about the symptoms that might suggest subsequent new retinal breaks or subsequent detachment associated with treated breaks. Several studies have suggested that patients have between a 5% and 10% chance of developing a new retinal tear in an eye that has previously undergone treatment. Such tears may occur remote from the area of treatment or may occur at the border of the treatment scar and normal retina. Therefore, any patient with new photopsias, substantially different floaters, or a peripheral field defect should be promptly reevaluated.

In the months following treatment (particularly cryopexy) the treated area may become more atrophic in appearance. If treatment was placed around the borders of a subclinical retinal detachment, the fluid within these borders will generally persist. The ophthalmologist should therefore not expect subretinal fluid within the borders of treatment to disappear entirely, although it may eventually do so.

Patients should be informed that treatment of retinal breaks is successful in about 95% of cases. Careful follow-up is necessary since 5% to 14% of eyes will subsequently develop new breaks in either eye.[17] Counseling regarding the symptoms of new tears and retinal detachment is mandatory. Patients should be instructed to cover the noninvolved eye regularly in the weeks following treatment and check their peripheral visual field. They should know that prompt management of a retinal tear may eliminate the need for retinal detachment surgery and that prompt management of a retinal detachment optimizes the chances for best final visual acuity. Additionally, patients should be informed of epiretinal membranes as a late complication of retinal tears—treated or untreated.

References

1. American Academy of Ophthalmology Preferred Practice Patterns Committee Retina Panel. Management of posterior vitreous detachment, retinal breaks, and lattice degeneration. San Francisco, 1998.
2. Byer NE. The natural history of asymptomatic retinal breaks. *Ophthalmology* 1982;89:1033.
3. Michelson IC, Stein R, Neuman E, et al. A national cooperative study in the prevention of retinal detachment. In: Pruet RC, Regan CDJ, eds. *Retina Congress.* New York: Appleton-Century-Crofts; 1972:661–667.
4. Benson WE, Grand G, Okun E. Aphakic retinal detachment. Management of the fellow eye. *Arch Ophthalmol* 1975;93:245–249.
5. Davis MD. Natural history of retinal breaks without detachment. *Arch Ophthalmol* 1974;92:183–194.
6. Merin S, Feiler V, Hyams S, et al. The fate of the fellow eye in retinal detachment. *Am J Ophthalmol* 1971;71:477–481.
7. Rowe JA, Erie JC, Gray DT, et al. Retinal detachment in Olmsted County, Minnesota 1976–1995. *Ophthalmology* 1999;106:154–159.
8. Tielsch JM, Legro MW, Cassard SD, et al. Risk factors for retinal detachment after cataract surgery. A population-based case-control study. *Ophthalmology* 1996;103:1537–1545.
9. The Eye Disease Case-Control Study Group. Risk factors for idiopathic rhegmatogenous retinal detachment. *Am J Epidemiol* 1993;137:749–757.
10. Burton TC. The influence of refractive error and lattice degeneration on the incidence of retinal detachment. *Trans Am Ophthalmol Soc* 1989;87:143–155.
11. Neumann E, Hymas S. Conservative management of retinal breaks. *Br J Ophthalmol* 1972;56:482.
12. Byer NE. Long-term natural history of lattice degeneration of the retina. *Ophthalmology* 1989;96:1396–1402.
13. Sigelman J. Vitreous base classification of retinal tears: clinical application. *Surv Ophthalmol* 1980;25:59.
14. Lincoff H, Kreissig I, Jakobiec F, et al. Remodeling of the cryosurgical adhesion. *Arch Ophthalmol* 1981;99:1845.
15. Roseman RL, Olk RJ, Arribas NP, et al. Limited retinal detachment: a retrospective analysis of treatment with transconjunctival retinocryopexy. *Ophthalmology* 1986;93:216.
16. Campochiaro PA, Kaden IH, Vidaurri-Leal J, et al. Cryotherapy enhances intravitreal dispersion of viable retinal pigment epithelial cells. *Arch Ophthalmol* 1985;103:434.
17. Smiddy WE, Flynn HW Jr, Nicholson DH, et al. Results and complications in treated retinal breaks. *Am J Ophthalmol* 1991;112:623–631.

5

Pneumatic Retinopexy

Paul E. Tornambe

This chapter emphasizes case selection, surgical technique, and complications of pneumatic retinopexy.

Pneumatic retinopexy, a term coined by George Hilton in 1985, uses a positioned intravitreal gas bubble to reattach the retina. Recent reports with this technique describe a single operation success rate of 83% and an overall success rate of 95%. These results are comparable to those of scleral buckling techniques.

The intraocular bubble works in two ways: (1) buoyancy—it pushes the retina against the retinal pigment epithelium, and (2) surface tension—it closes the retinal break, preventing liquid vitreous access to the subretinal space. The action of the retinal pigment epithelial (RPE) pump removes the remaining subretinal fluid, thereby reattaching the retina. The gas bubble reduces a retinal detachment to its primary component, a retinal tear. Once apposed to the eye wall, the retinal tear can be treated as one never associated with subretinal fluid, that is, with cryopexy or laser. Continued apposition of the bubble to the treated retina is maintained until a chorioretinal bond has formed. Once the edges of the break are sealed, eddy currents induced by eye movement will not dissect beneath the edges of the break and the retina will remain attached. The retinal detachment will recur if vitreous forces on the tear exceed the chorioretinal adhesion forces or if new breaks occur.

Patient Selection

The success of pneumatic retinopexy demands compliance. Patients selected for pneumatic retinopexy must be mentally and physically able to follow postoperative instructions. A senile or severely arthritic patient may be unable to maintain proper positioning. Patients with chronic obstructive pulmonary disease or congestive heart failure may be unable to assume the horizontal position necessary to close breaks at 3 or 9 o'clock. However, if medically compromised patients can tolerate the positioning, pneumatic retinopexy poses a lower surgical risk than conventional buckling surgery.

Ocular Considerations

Pneumatic retinopexy is an intraocular procedure. Attention should be directed toward lid hygiene, active hordeolums, or conjunctivitis. Eyes that have recently undergone intraocular surgery will have weakened sclera. A sudden rise in intraocular pressure could rupture a fresh wound, resulting in tissue prolapse. Eyes with severe glaucoma may not tolerate, even temporarily, elevated intraocular pressure. Such eyes should be treated with other techniques or softened sufficiently prior to injection of the gas bubble. Eyes with an unstable intraocular lens may not be good candidates for this procedure.

Retinal Considerations

Pneumatic retinopexy may be used to treat retinal detachments associated with retinal breaks, separated by up to 6 clock hours (180 degrees), located in the upper two-thirds of the fundus. Pneumatic retinopexy has been successfully used to treat retinal detachments associated with mild vitreous hemorrhage and posterior breaks, including macular holes. Although retinal breaks up to 2.5 clock hours in size have been successfully treated with pneumatic retinopexy, most retinal surgeons limit this technique to retinal breaks up to 1 clock hour in size. It may be used to treat retinal detachments associated with mild proliferative vitreoretinopathy (PVR) with star folds present in up to two quadrants of the retina (PVR C_2), as long as the star folds do not exert direct traction on the retinal breaks. This procedure should not be used for detachments associated with inferior breaks located between 4 and 8 o'clock. Eyes that demonstrate severe vitreoretinal traction, have extensive lattice degeneration (greater than 3 clock hours), or whose fellow eyes have sustained a giant retinal tear may not be good candidates. However, a very limber, motivated patient with a break at 5 or 7 o'clock may be adequately positioned and treated with pneumatic retinopexy.

Pneumatic retinopexy requires that all pathologic conditions be identified prior to injection of the gas bubble. The surgeon relinquishes the comfort of the operating room environment, where a relaxed, sedated patient with an open conjunctiva may undergo deep scleral depression. Inadequate visualization of the peripheral retina because of a poorly dilated pupil, media opacities, pseudophakia, or peripheral secondary capsular opacities may result in failure to detect a small break, resulting in failure of the retina to reattach.

Bubble Characteristics

The application of pneumatic retinopexy requires an understanding of intraocular gas expansion and geometry. The gas most frequently used is sulfur hexafluoride (SF_6). Perfluoropropane (C_3F_8 or PFP) is used occasionally. Both gases are inert, have poor solubility in water, and due to their high molecular weight, diffuse poorly out of the eye. Once the gas is injected into the vitreous cavity, osmotic forces draw in nitrogen and oxygen, expanding the volume of the gas bubble. A 0.3-cc injection of 100% SF6 will increase in size 2.5 times (i.e., to 0.75 cc) within 48 hours, while a 0.3-cc injection of 100% PFP will quadruple its volume (i.e., to 1.2 cc) in 72 hours. The greatest expansion of both gases occurs within the first 12–24 hours. The SF6 bubble usually persists 10–14 days, while the PFP bubble should last 4–6 weeks. A late rise in intraocular pressure owing to gas bubble expansion has not been reported. This is because the gas bubble acts as "internal tonography" and eyes with a relatively normal outflow facility compensate well. A potential problem might exist in eyes with glaucoma secondary to severely compromised outflow facility. These eyes may be treated with paracentesis as well as carbonic anhydrase inhibitors for a few days following the procedure.

Intraocular Bubble Geometry

In an emmetropic eye, a 0.3-cc bubble will subtend 1 clock hour of peripheral retinal arc. Much more gas is required to cover greater areas of retinal arc. A 0.8-cc bubble is necessary to subtend 2 clock hours at the equator, while a 2.4-cc bubble will subtend 6 clock hours (Figure 5-1).

Bubble Selection

Selection of the gas depends on the eye's facility for outflow and the size, location, number of retinal breaks, and existing vitreoretinal traction forces. A 0.1-cc injection of 100% PFP will expand to 0.4 cc over 3 days. This may be adequate to treat a small retinal break. However, if the break is larger, an initially small gas bubble may not close the break and could even pass through the retinal break into the subretinal space.

If there are several breaks several clock hours apart, a longer-acting bubble may be necessary to close the breaks sequentially or alternately. It is not necessary for a single bubble to treat all pathologic findings simultaneously (see section "Postoperative Care").

The degree of vitreoretinal traction must be considered. If significant vitreoretinal traction exists, bubble-break apposition may be necessary for several weeks, that is, until the chorioretinal scar has

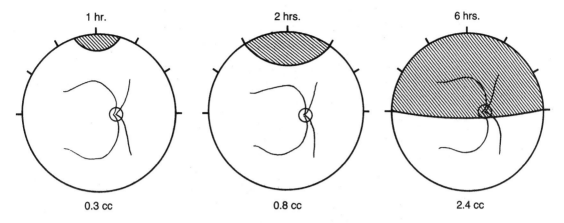

Figure 5-1. Bubble size versus arc of contact (emmetropic eye).

firmly evolved. Under such circumstances, a longer-acting bubble would be required. If the detachment is due to an atrophic or operculated hole with little residual vitreoretinal traction, a shorter-acting bubble is satisfactory.

Surgical Technique

The procedure may be done in the office examining chair, an outpatient facility, or rarely in the operating room (Table 5-1). Anesthesia is obtained by subconjunctival or peribulbar injection. Retrobulbar anesthesia is not necessary.

Light peripheral laser photocoagulation is applied to attached retina between the insertion of the vitreous base and ora serrata (Figure 5-2A). Cryopexy is applied to the tear(s) (Figures 5-2A and 5-3A) unless the "steamroller maneuver" is anticipated (see the following section). Cryopexy can be omitted and laser (delivered with the laser indirect ophthalmoscope using scleral depression) applied a few days later when the break has flattened (see Figure 5-2C). However, photocoagulation can be difficult in a partially gas-filled eye. Visibility is limited and care should be taken not to overtreat the retina with laser in areas in contact with gas. Without the "insulating effect" of the liquid vitreous, thermal burns can be excessive, resulting in retinal necrosis and hole formation.

A lid speculum is inserted and five drops of povidone-iodine (Betadine solution) are instilled and left in place for 3 minutes. The conjunctiva is then dried. A paracentesis (0.2–0.3 ml) is performed now, with a 27- or 30-gauge needle on a plungerless syringe, before gas bubble injection. The exact volume of gas (0.3–0.5 cc) to be injected is drawn through a millipore filter into a 1- or 3-ml syringe. With the patient supine, the head is turned 45 degrees to the opposite side so that the needle is perpendicular to the sclera (avoiding the lens) and points inferiorly toward the center of the globe and directly toward the floor. The sclera is perforated with a 27- or 30-gauge, $1/_2$-inch needle 3–4 mm from the limbus, preferably away from highly detached retina or large open retinal breaks. Do not inject where the pars plana epithelium is detached. Once the needle is in the vitreous cavity, it is pulled back so that only 2 mm of the tip is in the eye. The entire gas volume in the syringe is briskly injected. This permits injection of gas into the forming bubble so that a single bubble is created around the needle tip (Figure 5-3B). As the needle is withdrawn, a cotton-tipped applicator is placed over the perforation site and the patient's head is rotated to prevent gas from escaping through the sclerotomy. If the bubble is in the vitreous cavity, it will move to the most superior position in the eye. If the bubble is anterior to the anterior hyaloidal face, it will not move as the head is rotated and will appear oval. If it is under the retina, the bubble will look like a white, round pearl mobile in the subretinal space.

If multiple bubbles are present, the eye can be "flicked" with the index finger or a cotton-tipped applicator, which will force the bubbles to coalesce. The head should be turned 45 degrees to the opposite side so that the bubbles are positioned at the pars plana, away from the retinal breaks. That area

Table 5-1. Brief Summary of Protocol

A. Preoperative
1. Dilate pupil
2. Subconjunctival anesthesia

B. Operative
1. Patient supine.
2. Laser to periphral attached retina.
3. Transconjunctival cryopexy of retinal break; defer if steamroller technique is contemplated or if planned laser to peripheral retina when attached.
4. Place eyelid speculum.
5. Treat conjunctiva with 5 or 6 drops of povidone-iodine (Betadine solution) and wait 3 minutes.
6. Paracentesis.
7. Dry injection site 3–4 mm posterior to limbus with cotton-tipped applicator.
8. Briskly inject 0.3 cc sterile (Millipore filter) perfluoropropane or 0.5 cc sulfur hexafluoride gas with a $^1/_2$-inch 30-gauge needle through uppermost pars plana with needle pointing toward the floor.
9. Cover conjunctival perforation with sterile cotton-tipped applicator as needle is withdrawn, and turn head to move gas bubble away from injection site.
10. Observe central retinal artery. If the artery is closed, wait up to 10 minutes. If artery does not start to pulsate, use paracentesis.
11. Steamroller technique, if indicated, is performed now.
12. Continue to monitor central retinal artery and intraocular pressure (applanation) until the artery is patent and nonpulsatile. Apply cryopexy if steamroller technique was used.
13. Apply topical antibiotic and eye pad with arrow drawn for positioning.
14. Administer acetazolamide (Diamox) 250 mg four times daily if patient has glaucoma or will drive to a higher altitude, not exceeding 4,000 feet.

C. Postoperative
1. Instruct patient to position head so that the retinal break is uppermost (to position the gas bubble at the break site) for 16 hours a day.
2. Examine in office on first postoperative day. Discontinue use of eye pad.
3. Prescribe topical antibiotic and steroid solution four times daily.
4. Continue head positioning for 16 hours a day for 5 days. Patient may sleep on side for 8 hours each night but should not sleep on back.
5. Follow-up examinations at 1 and 3 days, and at 1, 2, 4, 8, 16, and 26 weeks.
6. Patient can return to work 3–4 weeks after surgery.

should then be "flicked" through the eyelid. If this is not successful, the patient should remain in a position to keep the small bubbles away from a large open retinal break for 24 hours. The multiple bubbles ("fish eggs") will usually coalesce over 12–24 hours. If a bubble passes under the retina, massaging it toward the break and back into the vitreous cavity can be tried with a scleral depressor. If this is not successful and the bubble is small, the eye should be observed closely. If the subretinal bubble is large, it should be removed.

Immediately after the injection, the central retinal artery is monitored. If the artery is closed, the time is noted with a stopwatch to measure the duration of closure. The absolute value of the intraocular pressure is not as important as the patency of the central retinal artery. In eyes containing gas, a 28-diopter lens provides the best view of the retina. Elevated intraocular pressure is usually not a problem after the intraocular injection of less than 0.5 cc of gas if a paracentesis has been performed. If a paracentesis has not been performed before gas bubble insertion, or more than 0.5 cc of gas is injected, immediate elevation of intraocular pressure to levels between 30 and 70 mm Hg is commonly observed, but pressure usually returns toward normal within 30–60 minutes. The intraocular pressure must be monitored by applanation tonometry, because Schiotz readings will be falsely low. If the central retinal artery remains nonpatent and nonpulsatile 10 minutes after the gas injection, a second paracentesis is done. Removal of a portion of the gas is rarely necessary. In phakic eyes or those with an intact posterior capsule, a limbal paracentesis is done. In aphakic eyes or those with an open posterior capsule, the needle is introduced through the pars plana and angled into the anterior chamber, where aqueous can be aspirated. This will avoid vitreous incarceration at the limbus. Once the intraocular pressure has returned to normal, even though the gas will later expand, a rise in intraocular pressure has not been noted.

If the detachment is so bullous that the central retinal artery cannot be visualized, the patient, in a sitting position, leans forward face down. The head is then rotated so that the gas bubble rolls nasally over the optic nerve, pushing the overhanging retina away. This will usually permit a view of the nerve and the central retinal artery.

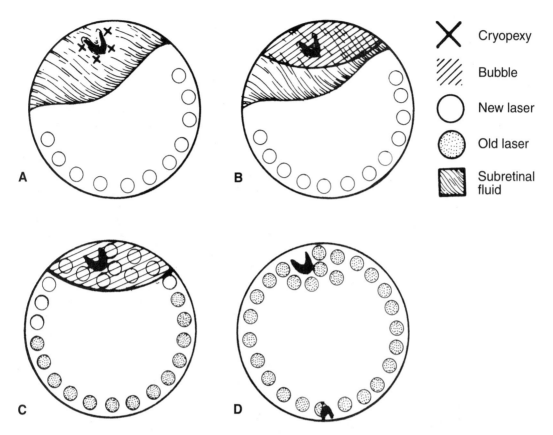

Figure 5-2. A, Laser photocoagulation is first applied to attached retina between the insertion of the vitreous base and ora. Avoid placing laser burns near detached retina. Light cryopexy is applied to the edges of the retinal break. **B,** After Betadine prep and paracentesis, intravitreal gas bubble is injected. **C,** 24–48 hours following gas injection, the retina attaches and laser is applied. **D,** If a new (or missed) retinal break develops after peripheral laser (in this case at 6 o'clock), the retina will not redetach.

The Steamroller Technique

The "steamroller" technique can be used to force subretinal fluid back into the vitreous cavity. The maneuver is recommended when the gas bubble might displace subretinal fluid beneath an attached macula or an attached inferior retinal break (Figure 5-4) or to prevent a macular fold (with a superior detachment and a large bubble). It can also be performed to "debulk" the overall size of the retinal detachment resulting in more rapid reattachment. The patient, in a sitting position, leans forward face down (Figure 5-5A). Over a 10-minute period, the patient's position is slowly changed from face down to a head position in which the retinal break is uppermost (Figure 5-5B). If this maneuver is anticipated, cryopexy should not be applied prior to gas

injection to minimize the chances of displacing viable RPE cells into the vitreous cavity. Although there may be a potential for displacing viable RPE cells into the vitreous cavity, the Pneumatic Retinopexy Clinical Trial did not show an increased incidence of macular pucker or PVR in eyes that had the steamroller maneuver performed.

A subconjunctival antibiotic may be administered near the injection site. The eye is patched and an arrow drawn on the patch to indicate the correct postoperative head position (i.e., the arrow should be aimed toward the ceiling). Alternatively the Escalon Pneumo Level can be used. This is an inexpensive (about $5) 1-inch, fluid-filled plastic disc containing a small air bubble with 12 clock hours printed on its face (Figure 5-6). It is affixed to the eye patch and the head positioned so the bubble

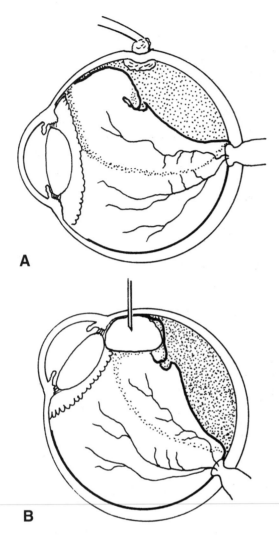

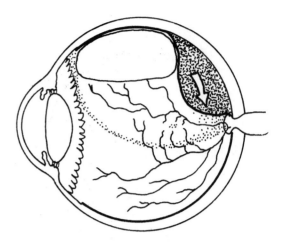

Figure 5-4. The gas bubble may displace subretinal fluid beneath the macula.

Figure 5-3. A, Cryopexy is applied to the retinal break. **B,** The needle is perpendicular to the floor so that the bubble forms around the needle tip avoiding "fish eggs."

lies over the desired clock hour. It greatly improves patient compliance and is particularly useful to aid positioning for breaks in the difficult 4 and 8 o'clock meridians. The patient and family are shown with a mirror the correct head posture to be maintained as long as possible for the first 24-hour period. A postoperative instruction sheet is given restating the procedure, medication, instructions, restrictions, and date for return visit. The patient is to use topical antibiotics four times daily, and prednisolone acetate drops four times daily for 10 days. For patients with glaucoma or those who will travel immediately by car to higher altitudes (no greater than 4,000 feet), carbonic anhydrase inhibitors are recommended for 3 days to minimize the chances of an excessive postoperative pressure rise. Air travel is avoided until the bubble completely resorbs. The patient is usually asked to return for a follow-up examination the following day.

Postoperative Care

It has been recommended that the patient be positioned so that the bubble is apposed to the retinal break for 16 hours a day for 3–5 days. Positioning duration depends upon the extent of vitreoretinal traction. For example, a retinal detachment secondary to a small, round break may be treated with bubble positioning until the break is flat. If there are no vitreoretinal traction forces, the RPE pump will hold the break apposed to the RPE while the chorioretinal adhesion forms. However, in cases with extensive vitreoretinal traction, bubble apposition may be necessary for longer periods of time.

It is not necessary for the bubble to be in contact with all breaks simultaneously. If multiple breaks exist, the patient is positioned so that the bubble closes the most superior breaks for the first few days. Then the patient is repositioned to close the remaining breaks. The patient can also be positioned alternately during the day so that all breaks are in contact with the bubble for a few hours each day.

Patients are examined on postoperative day 1. If the retina is flat, the patient returns in 1 week. If there

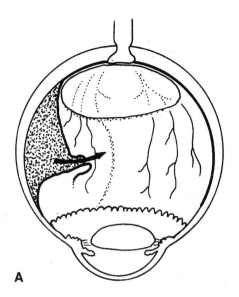 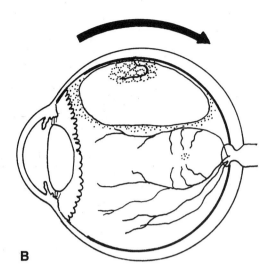

Figure 5-5. Steamroller maneuver. The patient is positioned face down (**A**), then slowly rotated so that the bubble rolls on the surface of the retina toward the retinal break (**B**), displacing subretinal fluid into the vitreous cavity.

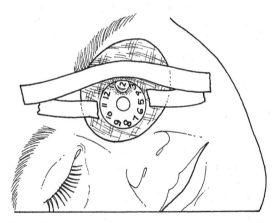

Figure 5-6. The Pneumo Level adheres to the eye patch and the patient is told to position his or her head so that the bubble is placed at a specific clock hour, in this case 2 o'clock.

has been little resorption of subretinal fluid after 24 hours, either an open or new break exists or the patient has not been positioned properly. A total bullous retinal detachment usually flattens completely within a few days. Sometimes thick, turbid subretinal fluid persists inferiorly and may take several weeks to resorb. As long as the macula is attached, these are managed conservatively. In some cases, isolated pockets of subretinal fluid in the midperiphery linger for weeks or months. These eyes should also be managed conservatively; the fluid eventually resorbs.

If the retina flattens within a few days, the patient is rechecked in 7–14 days. Use of topical antibiotics and steroid drops is maintained for 1–2 weeks. The patient is then seen on postoperative days 30, 60, 120, and 180. The patient is warned of the possibility of developing a new retinal break and told to notify the surgeon immediately if new flashes, floaters, or a curtain develop.

Patients are also instructed to contact the surgeon immediately if pain or loss of vision occurs, particularly within 24–72 hours after the intraocular injection, since this may represent the onset of endophthalmitis, which requires immediate treatment.

If the retina redetaches while gas is still in the eye secondary to a new break in the upper two-thirds of the fundus, the patient is repositioned to close the new break. If the bubble has absorbed or is not large enough, pneumatic retinopexy is repeated. If the break occurs inferiorly, a scleral buckling procedure is performed.

The patient may resume full activity 2–4 weeks after successful reattachment but is instructed not to fly or ascend to altitudes greater than 4,000 feet until the bubble completely resorbs. If the patient must undergo general anesthesia, the anesthesiologist should be warned of bubble expansion and induce the anesthesia appropriately (no nitrous oxide should be used).

Intraoperative Complications

The most serious intraoperative complication of pneumatic retinopexy is the subretinal injection of gas (Figure 5-7). If proper technique is followed (i.e., avoiding "fish eggs"), this complication can be avoided. If it does occur, the patient should be positioned and the eye massaged to displace the bubble back into the vitreous cavity. If the bubble is small, the patient can be managed conservatively. If a large bubble exists in the subretinal space, it must usually be surgically removed.

The complication of injection of gas anterior to the anterior hyaloid is usually easily treated by immediately reinserting the needle through the pars plana into the affected area with the barrel of the syringe removed. The gas will disperse passively. A new bubble can then be injected.

Damage to the lens is possible but should not occur if proper technique is used. Although a hemorrhage may occur at the pars plana injection site, it usually is not significant. Central retinal artery occlusion is possible and must always be considered. If the central retinal artery is closed for 10 minutes following the bubble injection, paracentesis is performed. The patient must not be discharged until the artery is patent and at least light perception documented. The intraocular pressure usually returns to the mid-20s within 1 hour following the injection of 0.3 cc of gas. A late rise in intraocular pressure has not been noted.

Displacement of subretinal fluid into the macula, macular folds or displacement of subretinal fluid inferiorly, elevating an inferior break, can be avoided if the steamroller technique is used.

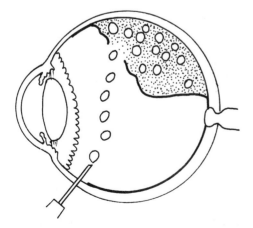

Figure 5-7. If the gas is injected from below, "fish eggs" will always result and may pass into the subretinal space.

Postoperative Complications

The most common postoperative complication of pneumatic retinopexy is failure of the retina to reattach owing to new or missed breaks. Failure of the retina to reattach within a few days usually indicates an open break. New breaks may occur immediately following the bubble injection, within the first few days, or even after several months. This may be due to increased traction or movement by the bubble, or contraction and separation of the vitreous. If the new break is not associated with subretinal fluid, it is treated with the laser or cryopexy. If the retina redetaches because of a new break in the upper two-thirds of the fundus, the pneumatic procedure can be repeated. Recent studies show that if a new retinal break occurs, the overall final anatomic and visual results with additional surgery are comparable to conventional primary buckling surgery.

One case of postoperative endophthalmitis to date has been reported following pneumatic retinopexy. There have been no reported cases of severe uveitis or choroidal detachment.

Case Selection and Surgical Technique

One operation success is strongly influenced by the phakic status of the eye, the number of retinal breaks, and the extent of the retinal detachment. A phakic quadrantic retinal detachment with one superior break carries a higher success rate than a total pseudophakic detachment with multiple retinal breaks. Light peripheral laser photocoagulation between the insertion of the vitreous base and ora serrata may also improve the single procedure success rate by prophylactically treating overlooked small breaks in attached retina, or by "pretreating" retina in an area where a new break later develops (see Figure 5-2D).

A Different Philosophy

The most important parameter to judge an ophthalmological procedure is vision. Visual acuity describes how one perceives the eye chart, vision describes how one perceives the environment. A 20/20 single operation surgical result might not be considered a success if objects are severely distorted, smaller or double. Pneumatic retinopexy does not change the shape of the eye nor interfere with the extraocular muscles; therefore it has the best chance to restore pre-detachment vision. Sight also returns more quickly following PR than scleral buckling, allowing patients to return to their normal lifestyle faster. Pneumatic retinopexy (an office procedure) is much less costly than scleral buckling (an OR procedure). Pneumatic retinopexy may have a lower single operation success rate than scleral buckling for some types of retinal detachments (pseudophakic, multiple breaks, more extensive areas involved). However, several authors have shown that a failed pneumatic attempt does not disadvantage the eye to ultimate anatomic and visual success. If final vision, patient morbidity, and cost are weighed against single operation success, pneumatic retinopexy remains a reasonable procedure to try first.

Conclusion

Pneumatic retinopexy is useful for the treatment of selected retinal detachments secondary to retinal breaks less than 1 clock hour in size located in the upper two-thirds of the fundus. It has also been successfully used to treat retinal detachments secondary to multiple retinal breaks separated by up to 180 degrees; giant tears; posterior breaks, including macular holes; and detachment associated with star folds that do not exert traction on the retinal breaks. Multiple breaks, pseudophakia, and subretinal fluid greater than 180 degrees are negative prognostic indicators that will lower the single operation success rate. However, a pneumatic failure does not disadvantage the eye in terms of a successful anatomic or visual outcome. Pneumatic retinopexy offers the advantages of minimal tissue trauma, minimal morbidity, rapid rehabilitation, and a significant reduction in cost.

Suggested Reading

Ambler JS, Meyers SM, Zegarra H, et al. Reoperations and visual results after failed pneumatic retinopexy. *Ophthalmology* 1990;97:786–790.

Boker T, Schmitt C, Mougharbel M. Results and prognostic factors in pneumatic retinopexy. *Ger J Ophthalmol* 1994;3:73–78.

Grizzard WS, Hilton GF, Hammer ME, et al. Pneumatic retinopexy failures. Cause, prevention, timing, and management. *Ophthalmology* 1995;102:929–936.

Hilton GF, Grizzard WS. Pneumatic retinopexy: a two-step operation without conjunctival incision. *Ophthalmology* 1986;93:626.

Hilton GF, Kelly NE, Tornambe PE, et al. Pneumatic retinopexy: a collaborative report of the first 100 cases. *Ophthalmology* 1987;94(4):307.

Lincoff A, Half D, Liggett P, et al. Intravitreal expansion of perfluorocarbon gases. *Arch Ophthalmol* 1980;98:1646.

Lincoff H, Coleman J, Kressig I, et al. The perfluorocarbon gases in the treatment of retinal detachment. *Ophthalmology* 1983;90:546.

Poliner LS, Grand MG, Shock LH, et al. New retinal detachment following pneumatic retinopexy. *Ophthalmology* 1987;94(4):315.

Tornambe PE. Pneumatic retinopexy. *Surv Ophthalmol* 1988;32:270.

Tornambe PE. Pneumatic retinopexy: The evolution of case selection and surgical technique—A twelve-year study of 302 eyes. *Transactions of the American Ophthalmological Society,* Vol. XCV, December 1997.

Tornambe PE, Grizzard WS, eds. *Pneumatic Retinopexy: A Clinical Symposium.* Westport, CT: Greenwood Publishing; 1989.

Tornambe PE, Hilton GF. The pneumatic retinopexy study group. Pneumatic retinopexy—A multicenter randomized controlled clinical trial comparing pneumatic retinopexy with scleral buckling. *Ophthalmol* 1989;96:772–783.

Tornambe PE, Hilton GF. The pneumatic retinopexy study group. Pneumatic retinopexy—A two-year follow-up study of the multicenter clinical trial comparing pneumatic retinopexy with scleral buckling. *Ophthalmol* 1991;98:1115–1123.

Tornambe PE, Hilton GF, Kelly NE, et al. Expanded indications for pneumatic retinopathy. *Ophthalmol* 1988;95:597.

6

Anesthesia for Vitreoretinal Surgery

W. Sanderson Grizzard

In the last edition of this book I predicted that "retinal surgeons will also be doing more local and outpatient surgery." This certainly is true. Today, I do more than 90% of my surgery under local anesthesia. I have had one inpatient in 2 years. Improvements in general anesthesia and local sedation have aided in this transition to outpatient surgery. Patients usually wake up quickly and quietly from modern general anesthesia. Patients do better at home following surgery where they sleep in their own bed and are cared for by their family. Diabetic patients are usually able to manage their own insulin and medical problems at home.

There are two basic approaches: (1) general endotrachial anesthesia and (2) local infiltration or nerve block anesthesia. The two techniques blur in clinical practice. Patients receiving local anesthesia are often sedated, and patients receiving general anesthesia are often given periocular injections of local anesthetic to decrease the required depth of general anesthesia and to aid with post-operative pain management. The selection of anesthetic technique is difficult for the retinal surgeon, because of the emergent nature of the surgery and the consultative nature of a retina practice. Often the patient is referred away from his usual medical care provider and the patient's medical condition is not well known to the surgeon.

Techniques of local anesthetic injection have changed over the last 10 years. The Atkinson technique ("looking up and in") has fallen into disfavor. Peribulbar anesthesia involving larger volumes of anesthetic injected away from the globe is now the most commonly used approach. Minimalist techniques involving topical anesthesia, subconjunctival injections, and posterior irrigation have been proposed to diminish the risk of local anesthesia. Bupivacaine (Marcaine) is now the most commonly used agent allowing blocks of much longer duration. New drugs for general anesthesia and new monitoring devices have, likewise, become available.

Patient Selection

No one anesthetic technique is right for every patient or every operation. Over the years I have developed prejudices about which patients will do well with local anesthesia or local anesthesia supplemented by intravenous sedation. I have developed a scoring system to select patients for local anesthesia (Table 6-1). Patients with a score of greater than three usually do better with general anesthesia or general anesthesia supplemented with local injection.

Numerous factors influence the selection of an anesthetic. Which procedure is being done? How cooperative is the patient? How familiar is the surgeon with the operating environment and the operating room personnel? As more experience is acquired, it is possible to raise your threshold score. After a few bad experiences, however, it may be wise to lower it for a while.

Table 6-1. Scoring System to Select Patients for Local Versus General Anesthesia

Factor	Points
Procedure	
Pneumatic retinopexy	0
Primary scleral buckling	1
"Easy" revision of buckling	2
Difficult revision of buckling	3
Simple vitrectomy	2
Vitrectomy with preretinal membrane removal or macular hole surgery	2
Vitrectomy for endophthalmitis	3
Vitrectomy for proliferative vitreoretinopathy (PVR) or proliferative diabetic retinopathy	4
Patient Factors	
Under age 60	1
Under age 40	2
Male	1
Trouble with previous local eye surgery	2
Could not tolerate retinal examination with scleral depression	2
High myopia	2
Prefers general anesthetic	2
Severe cardiac or respiratory disease	–2
Patient just ate	–2
Operating Room Conditions	
Inexperienced crew in operating room	1
Excellent anesthetic department	1
Operating at unfamiliar hospital	1
Teaching situation	2
Surgeon just out of fellowship	2

Vitrectomy and primary scleral buckle procedures can usually be done with local anesthesia. Vitrectomies can be done with local anesthesia more easily than a scleral buckle. Complex vitrectomies combined with scleral buckling may need general anesthesia or general anesthesia supplemented by periocular anesthetic injection. Endophthalmitis is a special situation because it is difficult to get a good block if there is orbital inflammation (see the section in this chapter on pharmacology). If only a tap with injection of antibiotics is necessary local injection may be adequate. If vitrectomy is going to be part of the management strategy, I find that general anesthesia is frequently necessary and should be available if a local block fails.

The most important "patient factors" are age and the ability to undergo a good retinal examination in the office. Young patients who are squeamish during scleral depression are best treated under general anesthesia. Older patients who have previously had cataract surgery are excellent candidates for local anesthesia.

The environment of the operating room is also important in selecting which technique to use. Surgeons who are just out of training or who are in a new hospital may prefer to have the patient asleep. Operating room personnel who respond, "What's that?" when asked for every instrument can make an experienced surgeon wish that the patient were asleep. It is also much easier to teach when the patient is asleep!

In summary, patient selection for local anesthesia is an art. We have all found ourselves in a situation where we wished we had made the other choice. Table 6-1 and a little experience will, it is hoped, minimize those situations.

Anatomy

To safely provide regional anesthesia for ocular surgery, it is necessary to have a thorough knowledge of orbital and periorbital anatomy and to understand the anatomic changes that take place during ocular movement.

The anterior orbit is occupied by the eye, which geometrically is a modified sphere or two merged spheres, one in front of the other. The emmetropic eye has an anteroposterior diameter of approximately 24 mm and a vertical diameter of 23 mm. In myopia, the eye is larger with a more elongated, ovoid shape. In eyes with more than 4-diopters of myopia, the axial length varies from 26.7 to 31.0 mm. A line joining the medial and lateral orbital margins will have a third of the eye anterior to it. The lateral orbital rim is more posterior than the medial orbital rim. The equator of the eye is generally at, or slightly anterior to, the lateral orbital rim. The eye is closer to the roof of the orbit than to the floor and the frontal bone overhangs the eye, making the inferotemporal approach the most open access to the retrobulbar space.

The concept of a well-defined muscle cone formed anteriorly by the coronal circumference of the eye and posteriorly by the rectus muscles with a well-developed intermuscular septum has been shown to be not only a simplification but inaccurate. Anteriorly, there are well-formed connective tissue septa connecting the ocular muscles; posteriorly, however, the intermuscular septum becomes less well defined and more complex connective tissue septa appear. Two poorly septated areas in the orbit, one lateral to the optic nerve and the other above the superior ophthalmic vein hammock, account for the high success rate of both retrobulbar and peribulbar anesthesia. The lateral rectus and inferior rectus muscles are in close proximity to the orbital wall. A large extraconal space does not exist either temporally or inferiorly.

The optic nerve, the cranial motor and sensory nerves, and the arterial circulation to the eye enter the orbit posteriorly. Although a well-defined annulus of Zinn or common tendinous ring does not exist, it is convenient to think of three posterior openings: (1) the superior orbital fissure superior to the tendinous insertions, (2) the superior orbital fissure inferior to the tendinous insertion, and (3) the optic foramen.

Through the optic foramen and the optic canal that lie within the lesser wing of the sphenoid bone (SB) pass the optic nerve (ON) and the ophthalmic artery (OA) (Figure 6-1). After the optic nerve enters the orbit through the optic canal, it courses anteriorly for about 30 mm before entering the eye. The distance from the optic foramen to the temporal orbital rim has been evaluated and found to be extremely variable. Although the mean is 50–51 mm, the range extends from 45–58 mm.

Accompanying the optic nerve is the main vascular supply to the orbit and eye, the ophthalmic artery. This artery is the first intracranial branch of the carotid artery, sharing the dural sheath with the optic nerve while in the optic canal. On exiting the canal, it courses laterally giving off the central retinal artery and then crosses superiorly over the optic nerve giving off its branches, the lacrimal artery, the posterior ethmoidal artery, the long and short posterior ciliary arteries, and the branches that course anteriorly.

The sensory nerves to the eye, orbit, and lids are branches of the trigeminal nerve. The lacrimal nerve (LN), the frontal nerve (FN), and the nasociliary nerve (NCN) are branches of the ophthalmic division and enter the orbit through the superior orbital fissure (superior to the tendinous insertions), as shown in Figure 6-1. The tendinous ring is not well formed, particularly temporally, where the motor and sensory nerves enter the orbit.

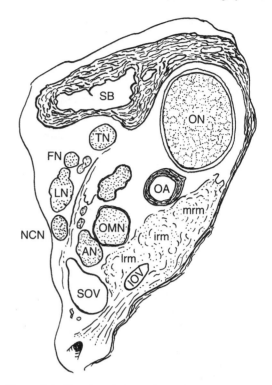

Figure 6-1. SB, sphenoid bone; ON, optic nerve; TN, trochlear nerve; FN, frontal nerve; LN, lacrimal nerve; OA, ophthalmic artery; NCN, nasociliary nerve; AN, abducens nerve; OMN, oculomotor nerve; SOV, superior ophthalmic vein; IOV, inferior ophthalmic vein; lrm, lateral rectus muscle; irm, inferior rectus muscle; mrm, medial rectus muscle.

The frontal nerve and lacrimal nerve are the most superior structures in the orbit and are just below the periorbita. The frontal nerve courses anteriorly and medially, branching into the supratrochlear (STN) and the supraorbital nerve (SON), as shown in Figure 6-2. The supratrochlear nerve courses anteriorly, exiting the orbit just above the trochlea of the superior oblique muscle; it supplies the skin and conjunctiva of the medial part of the upper lid and a small part of the skin of the upper forehead and nose (Figure 6-3). The supraorbital nerve courses above the levator muscle anteriorly, exiting the orbit through the supraorbital notch. The supraorbital nerve supplies the forehead and scalp and the skin and conjunctiva of the middle upper eyelid. The LN courses laterally, superior to the lateral rectus muscle on its way to the lacrimal gland. It innervates the lacrimal gland and the conjunctiva and skin of the temporal part of the upper and lower lids.

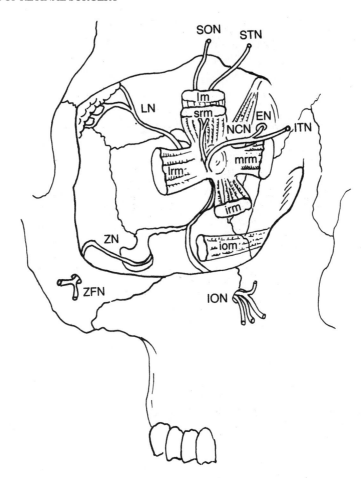

Figure 6-2. LN, lacrimal nerve; ZN, zygomatic nerve; ZFN, zygomatic facial nerve; ION, infraorbital nerve; SON, supraorbital nerve; STN, supratrochlear nerve; NCN, nasociliary nerve; EN, ethmoidal nerve; srm, superior rectus muscle; som, superior oblique muscle; mrm, medial rectus muscle; irm, inferior rectus muscle; iom, inferior oblique muscle; lrm, lateral rectus muscle; lm, levator muscle.

The NCN enters the orbit with the other branches of the ophthalmic division (Figure 6-1). It then enters the muscle cone and runs above the optic nerve, giving off a branch to the ciliary ganglion and the two long, posterior ciliary nerves (Figure 6-2). It then courses nasally to the medial orbital wall, giving off the ethmoidal nerves (EN) and becoming the infratrochlear nerve (ITN). The ciliary ganglion lies well back in the orbit, lateral to the optic nerve, and receives the preganglionic, parasympathetic fibers from the inferior branch of the oculomotor nerve. The short ciliary nerves are given off by the ciliary ganglion and enter the globe posteriorly around the optic nerve. The afferent sensory supply from the globe courses through the short and long ciliary nerves, as do the sympathetic and parasympathetic

innervation to the pupil. Good anesthesia to the nasociliary nerve, therefore, results in pupillary dilation from parasympathetic blockage.

The maxillary division of the trigeminal nerve exits the middle cranial fossa through the foramen rotundum and transverses the pterygopalatine fossa, where it gives off the posterior superior alveolar nerve to the posterior superior teeth. It then gives off the zygomatic nerve (ZN) and becomes the infraorbital nerve (ION) as it enters the orbit through the infraorbital fissure and travels through the maxillary bone in the infraorbital canal to exit the skull through the infraorbital foramen. The ZN travels along the infraorbital fissure and gives off two branches, the zygomaticofacial (ZFN) and the zygomaticotemporal (ZTN) nerves, which supply afferent sensory

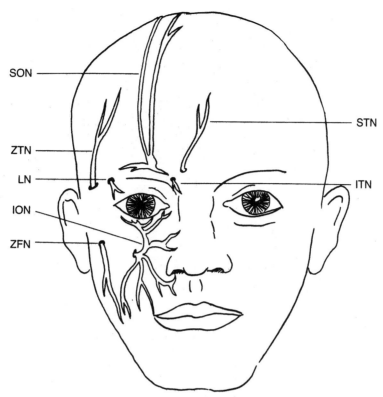

Figure 6-3. SON, supraorbital nerve; ZTN, zygomatic temporal nerve; LN, lacrimal nerve; ION, infraorbital nerve; ZFN, zygomatic facial nerve; STN, supratrochlear nerve; ITN, infratrochlear nerve.

nerves to the lateral aspect of the upper and lower lid and conjunctiva. There are also deep pain fibers in the inferotemporal aspect of the orbit supplied by these nerves, which must be blocked for scleral buckling procedures (see Figure 6-2).

Inferiorly and nasally in the superior orbital fissure, the upper and lower divisions of the oculomotor nerve (OMN) (motor nerves to the levator, superior rectus [srm], medial rectus [mrm], inferior rectus [irm], and inferior oblique, and the abducens nerve (AN)—motor nerve to the lateral rectus [lrm]) enter the orbit from the middle cranial fossa (see Figure 6-1). The trochlear nerve enters superiorly in the superior orbital fissure (see Figure 6-1).

During changes in gaze, the structures within the orbit undergo rapid changes. The eye, if it is spherical, rotates around a central point but does not have significant lateral or vertical motion. The rectus muscles are fixed posteriorly by their tendinous origins and anteriorly by their functional insertion in the coronal, equatorial plane of the eye. The concept of "presenting the cone" by having the patient look away from the needle is a geometric impossibility. The position of the cone does not move. What does move are the structures within the cone. A 30-mm intraorbital portion of the optic nerve is needed to accommodate eye movement. The other intraconal structures also must move because they are held in place relative to the optic nerve by a three dimensional net of connective tissue.

The Atkinson position for retrobulbar injection (i.e., "up and in") causes the optic nerve to be brought inferotemporally and held in a position directly in the path of the needle (Figure 6-4A). Likewise, if the eye is not spherical but ovoid, as occurs in myopia, the posterior pole of the eye moves inferiorly toward the oncoming needle. It is much safer to maintain the eye in the primary gaze position and direct the needle to a point behind the macula (Figure 6-4B). If one is injecting superiorly, it is unwise to have the patient look down for the same reason. The ciliary ganglion and the nasociliary nerve sit superiorly near the optic nerve and move with it. This accounts for the higher success

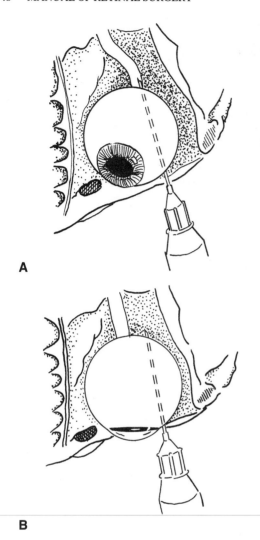

A

B

Figure 6-4. A, Atkinson position for the retrobulbar injection ("up and in") endangers the optic nerve. **B,** Maintaining the eye in primary gaze position is safer.

rate when using the Atkinson technique, but the optic nerve position accounts for the attendant high incidence of optic nerve complications.

It is important to remember that the brain stem sits just behind the orbit and is separated from it by the sphenoid bone and dura. The optic canal and the supraorbital foramen allow passage of arteries, veins, and nerves from the middle cranial fossa to the orbit. The barrier between the brain and the orbit is not impermeable. If the anesthetic passes through the dura of the optic nerve such that all vision (no light perception) is lost, the anesthetic also will pass through the dura into the brain stem.

Needle perforation of the optic nerve is not necessary for central nervous system effects.

Pharmacology

Local anesthetics are drugs that interrupt nerve conduction by interfering with the propagation of the nerve action potential. Nerves at rest are polarized with sodium ions in excess outside the membrane. As the membrane is stimulated there is an influx of sodium into the cell and an outflow of potassium. The shift in ions causes formation of an action potential of 50–90 mV that is propagated along the neuron.

Local anesthetics interfere with this excitation process by displacing calcium ions from their binding sites, so that changes in membrane permeability do not occur and the membrane is not depolarized. Thus, the threshold potential cannot then be reached and there is no propagation of the impulse.

Local anesthetics are grouped into two categories by chemical structure: the esters and the amines. The esters (such as procaine) were commonly used before 1940 but have been largely replaced by the amines (such as lidocaine). Amine salts are more stable and water soluble than the bases, so the local anesthetics we use come in solution as salts. To be active they must revert to their uncharged form—the base. The percentage of the base form is determined by the pH of the tissue and the pKa of the salt. In inflamed tissue, the pH is lower so that there is less bioactive form available in the tissue. Repeated injection into the tissue to augment the block further lowers the pH, making matters worse. In severely inflamed tissue, such as occurs in endophthalmitis, it is best to be prepared to convert to general anesthesia. Etidocaine (Duranest) may be the best drug for this situation since its pKa is 7.7 and 33% of it is in the active form at pH 7.4.

Table 6-2 briefly reviews concentrations, dosages, and duration of action of commonly used ophthalmic drugs. Lidocaine (Xylocaine), the most commonly used local anesthetic, has a duration of action that is marginally adequate for retinal procedures. Bupivacaine (Marcaine) has become the standard because of its longer duration of action. Because it has a slower onset of effective motor and sensory block, many surgeons mix it with lidocaine to get a more rapid onset of action. Etidocaine is

Table 6-2. Commonly Used Ophthalmic Anesthetics

Drug	Concentration (%)	Maximum Dose (mg)	Maximum Volume (ml)	Duration of Block (min)
Lidocaine	1	300	30	90
(Xylocaine)	2	300	15	
	4	200	5	
Bupivacaine	0.5	150	30	180
(Marcaine)	0.75	30	4[a]	
Etidocaine	1 or 1.5	60	4[a]	180
(Duranest)				

[a] Denotes specific retrobulbar dosage recommendation by drug manufacturers; others are for peripheral nerve block.

less popular because of its prolonged motor block and increased cost, but it may offer some advantages, such as decreasing postoperative eye movement and being more effective in low pH environments.

Bupivacaine has been implicated as causing respiratory arrest when used for retrobulbar injections. In my opinion, it is no more dangerous at the dosages used in ophthalmology than are other anesthetics. The cases of cardiac arrest caused by bupivacaine during epidural anesthesia involved much larger volumes of anesthetic, which may have a direct cardiac effect.

Epinephrine can be added to local anesthetics to prolong their action by 50–100%. This is necessary when performing scleral buckling with lidocaine, but is not generally necessary when using bupivacaine and etidocaine. I prefer not to use it because of potential systemic and local reactions. Hyaluronidase (Wydase) is also frequently added to retrobulbar injections to promote a more rapid diffusion of anesthetic. This practice has fallen into disuse in all other branches of surgery and I have discontinued using it without any noticeable effect. I know of one patient who had a severe allergic reaction to Hyaluronidase and lost the eye.

Needles

I use a sharp, 27-gauge, $1\frac{1}{4}$-inch (32-mm) disposable needle. There is controversy concerning which needle is best. I believe that blunt needles cause much greater pain and are not safer than sharp needles. Sharpness is determined by many factors; the angle of the tip, the angle of the bevel face, the

number of facets on the bevel edge, and the thickness of the shaft (Figure 6-5).

Long needles, both the $1\frac{1}{2}$-inch (37-mm) needle and particularly the 2-inch (50-mm) needle give better blocks because they reach into the apex of the orbit, where the nerves and vessels are crowded together. This same advantage becomes a disadvantage because damage to the apical structures, orbital hemorrhage, and inadvertent injection into the optic nerve and brain stem are more likely with longer needles.

Many complications of retrobulbar injection have been attributed to the use of a sharp needle. In my opinion, most of these complications were due

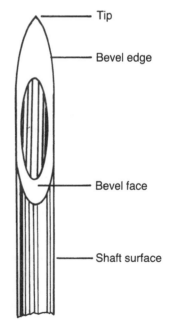

Figure 6-5. Components of a needle.

to inappropriate technique (the Atkinson position of gaze) or long needles. Ocular penetration, optic nerve penetration, retrobulbar hemorrhage, and central nervous system effects have all occurred following the use of a blunt needle.

The theoretical advantage of a blunt needle is that it requires more force to penetrate a tissue; therefore, it will be easier to detect the resistance of sclera or optic nerve dura. The other supposed advantage is that the optic nerve and sclera will slide away from the oncoming blunt needle. Unfortunately, this increased resistance caused by the blunt needle is more difficult to detect because of the greater preload caused by the blunt needle (Weber-Fechner law). The fibrous framework of the orbit that attaches to the eye and optic nerve does not allow them to move out of the way, as has been proposed. The true situation in the orbit is analogous to a full pickle jar, not a nearly empty one.

The main advantage of a sharp needle is that heavy premedication is not necessary in most patients. This is important if there is no anesthesiologist available. I also believe that if one uses a sharp needle one will be more careful when placing the needle and doing the block. The most dangerous situation is a nonophthalmologist with a long, blunt needle who thinks ocular penetration and optic nerve damage are impossible.

Premedication and Monitoring

I prefer that my patients not receive heavy premedication before the anesthetic injection. I particularly do not like to have the patients put to sleep with short-acting barbiturates or propofol (Diprivan) so that I can give them a local injection. A knowledgeable, competent, and reassuring staff is the best preoperative sedation. If the patient is particularly anxious, mild preoperative medication may be helpful. With patients experiencing severe anxiety, it may be better to consider general anesthesia. Intravenous midazolam (Versed) or propofol (Diprivan) can be given for sedation if necessary but the patient must be carefully monitored. Its use has been associated with respiratory depression and cardiac arrest. I always consider it wise to have trained anesthesia personnel monitor the patient during surgery because of the potential for cardiac and respiratory arrest.

Monitoring devices available should include a blood pressure cuff, a cardiac monitor, and a device for measuring oxygen saturation (pulse oximeter). The pulse oximeter is ideal for detecting respiratory insufficiency before it results in cardiac arrhythmia or arrest. Unfortunately, in awake patients it can sometimes be difficult to keep it functioning properly. I do believe that the patient should be observed closely following a retrobulbar injection. Electronic monitoring is not necessarily indicated, but the patient should not be left unattended.

Technique

Several different anesthetic "cocktails" are in current use and come and go in popularity. I prefer to use as simple a mixture as possible. Table 6-3 reflects my recent experience. I generally use bupivacaine or bupivacaine mixed with lidocaine. The motor block may be delayed with bupivacaine alone, but the sensory block is usually adequate for retinal surgery. The postoperative analgesia from bupivacaine is very helpful, particularly for outpatient surgery. The drugs are inexpensive.

Start the block by raising a skin weal with a small amount of the anesthetic mixture and then follow by doing a retrobulbar injection using 4–5 ml of the anesthetic with the eye in primary gaze. A sharp $1^{1}/_{4}$-inch (32-mm), 27-gauge needle is introduced through the skin weal immediately above the inferior orbital rim between the temporal limbus and the lateral canthus with the intention of avoiding the recti muscles (Figure 6-6, point A). Some surgeons at this point place a finger between the globe and the inferotemporal rim of the orbit to "push" the globe out of harms way. When the needle is advanced beyond the equator of the globe, it is directed toward an imaginary point behind the macula (see Figure 6-6, point A). Remember to inject very slowly to avoid discomfort to the patient and to prevent a sudden intravascular bolus if the needle happens to be within a vessel. Aspiration before injection to rule out intravascular placement of the needle is an added safety precaution. Next, partially withdraw the needle and inject an additional 2 ml with the needle 1–2 cm below the skin directed straight posteriorly. This is particularly important when doing a scleral buckle, but unnecessary for other procedures. Next, I instill topical

Table 6-3. Author's Personal Experience with Certain Anesthetics for Use in Retinal Surgery

Anesthetic	Advantages	Disadvantages
Lidocaine 2% (Xylocaine)	Familiar drug Prompt analgesia and motor block Established safety	Short duration of action Needs epinephrine for retinal surgery
Bupivacaine 0.75% (Marcaine)	Adequate speed of onset for anesthesia Long duration of action Good postoperative analgesia	More than 4 ml exceeds dose recommended by manufacturer Motor block delayed Reports of respiratory arrest
Bupivacaine 0.5% (Marcaine)	Long duration of action Good postoperative analgesia Possibly safer than 0.75% bupivacaine	Onset of anesthesia delayed Poor motor block
Bupivacaine 0.75% mixed with 2% lidocaine or 4% lidocaine	Prompt analgesia and motor block Good postoperative analgesias	Practice not recommended by manufaturer High incidence of brain stem anesthesia in one report (Wittpenn, et al.; 1986)

anesthetic into the conjunctival sac and then place digital pressure on the eye. Next, I remove the $1^1/_4$-inch needle from the syringe and using a $^5/_8$-inch needle place the needle through the caruncle directed superiorly at a 45-degree angle, away from the globe (Figure 6-6, point B). For this part of the injection a right-handed surgeon should stand to the right of the supine patient for both the right and left eye. Left-handed surgeons should stand to the left for both eyes. Penetrate to the hub of the needle and inject 3 ml slowly. You can see the anesthetic spread along the upper lid. This approach avoids the vascular superior orbit and also avoids injecting supero-temporally where the superior orbital rim overhangs the eye and makes safe injection difficult. This approach blocks the frontal and supratrochlear nerves.

I then place a Honan balloon to soften the eye and spread the anesthetic. If a soft eye is not critical, a few minutes of ocular massage spreads the anesthetic. No lid block is necessary; this can be the most painful part of the procedure.

After the eye is draped, a lid speculum is inserted. I then inject a small amount of 0.5% bupivacaine (Marcaine), with or without epinephrine, under the conjunctiva. This helps with dissection and gives good anesthesia to the conjunctiva initially and more importantly at the end of the surgery when often the patient feels pain during closure. If there is pain with the posterior dissection, local

infiltration in that quadrant with 0.5% bupivacaine (Marcaine) often solves the problem. The blunt, curved irrigation cannula can be used to irrigate anesthetic solution behind the eye (in each of the quadrants). If the discomfort comes from manipulating the muscles, a posterior injection may be necessary. Be careful doing these injections because the muscle cone narrows abruptly posterior to the globe.

Complications

The advantage of using local anesthesia for ocular surgery and, in particular, retinal surgery is that patients have so few serious complications. As with any other surgical intervention, however, certain problems do arise.

Respiratory arrest and death have been reported following retrobulbar injection and have been attributed to an allergic or idiosyncratic reaction to the drug, systemic toxicity from intravascular injection, or a brain stem injection through the optic nerve and optic foramen. Many of these cases have been the result of retinal surgery. The most probable mechanism is the latter, which can be avoided by using proper technique and shorter needles.

Retinal vascular problems and unexplained optic atrophy following retinal surgery generally are blamed on the surgery itself and not the anesthetic.

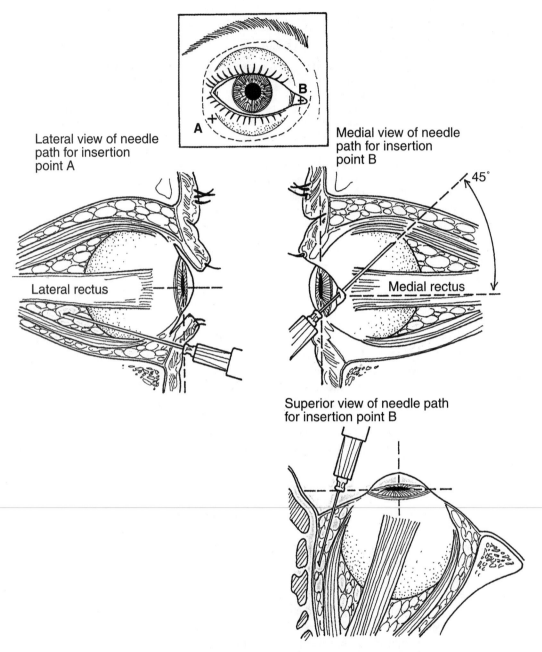

Figure 6-6. Retrobulbar injection. Start the block by raising a skin weal with a small amount of the anesthetic mixture and then follow with the retrobulbar injection using 4–5 ml of the anesthetic with the eye in primary gaze. A sharp $1\frac{1}{4}$-inch (32-mm), 27-gauge needle is introduced through the skin weal immediately above the inferior orbital rim between the temporal limbus and the lateral canthus (point A). When the needle is advanced beyond the equator of the globe, it is directed toward an imaginary point behind the macula. Next, partially withdraw the needle and inject an additional 2 ml with the needle 1–2 cm below the skin directed straight posteriorly. This is particularly important when doing a scleral buckle but unnecessary for other procedures. Next I instill topical anesthetic into the conjunctival sac and then place digital pressure on the eye. I then remove the $1\frac{1}{4}$-inch needle from the syringe and using a $\frac{5}{8}$-inch needle place the needle through the caruncle directed superiorly at a 45-degree angle superiorly, away from the globe (point B). Penetrate to the hub of the needle and inject 3 ml slowly. You can see the anesthetic spread along the upper lid. This approach avoids the vascular superior orbit and also avoids injecting superiorly where the superior orbital rim overhangs the eye and makes safe injection difficult.

When these problems occur following pterygium removal or radial keratotomy, however, it is difficult to ignore the possible contribution of the retrobulbar injection. Avoiding optic nerve penetration is easy if one remembers to have the patient maintain primary gaze and if one uses a short needle. If retinal vascular occlusion occurs, evaluation of the optic nerve by computed tomography is necessary to rule out intranerve-sheath hemorrhage. If an intranerve-sheath hemorrhage or a dilated nerve is found, decompression of the optic nerve may be beneficial.

Ocular penetration has also been reported following retrobulbar and peribulbar injections. It is more likely to occur in myopic eyes because they are larger, have thinner sclera, and are ovoid. The ovoid eye causes problems because, in the traditional Atkinson position, the posterior pole of the eye is brought into the path of the oncoming needle. Therefore, in highly myopic and large eyes, consideration should be given to using general anesthesia. Blunt needles have been recommended in this setting; however, the thin sclera further limits the surgeon's ability to feel ocular penetration.

Intraocular injection of lidocaine has occurred and is not itself toxic to the retina. Intracameral xylocaine is now frequently used in cataract surgery. In one case of inadvertent intraocular injection, there was initial loss of light perception with full visual recovery within 16 hours. If this happens, the eye should be softened and observed for retinal vascular problems. If an ocular perforation (entry and exit wound) occurs, the planned retinal surgery should be carried out to fix the retinal detachment and to treat the newly made retinal holes. If vitreous hemorrhage prevents adequate visualization, or if there are posterior breaks, vitrectomy may be necessary.

Retrobulbar hemorrhage is the most common problem following retrobulbar injection. If one uses shorter needles and primary gaze, the incidence of this problem is low because the highly vascular orbital apex is avoided.

General Anesthesia

The safety of anesthesia and our ability to monitor patients have improved greatly. Undue fear of anesthetic risk is no longer appropriate when one works with a well-trained anesthesiologist. In addition to the use of stethoscopes, cardiac monitors, and blood pressure cuffs, instruments to measure expiratory carbon dioxide, oxygen saturation, core body temperature, and arterial pulse pressures can be routinely used. This helps to minimize the risk of anesthetic accidents.

There still remains the risk of allergic and idiosyncratic reactions to anesthetic agents and the problem of medically unstable patients. Patients who have recently experienced myocardial infarction present a special problem when faced with the need for a general anesthetic. These patients should be managed with local anesthesia. Close consultation with the patient, the patient's physician, and the anesthesiologist is critical in this setting. Sometimes even urgent, sight-saving surgery should be delayed or canceled.

Another special problem that retinal surgeons face with the use of general anesthesia is the effect that inspired anesthetic gas mixtures have on the volume of gas bubbles and the intraocular pressure of the eye. The problem exists in three parts:

1. What happens during anesthetic induction to eyes that already have a gas bubble in them?
2. What is the effect on a gas bubble placed during surgery?
3. What happens to the gas bubble in the eye after the anesthetic gases are discontinued?

A basic knowledge of the physics of gases is necessary to understand what happens and how to deal with it.

Gases in body cavities try to establish equilibrium with the gases in solution in the blood, so that the same gas mixture exists in the body cavity as in the blood. This is the "second gas effect." Gas moves in both directions to establish this equilibrium. The speed with which this occurs depends on the molecular weight, the diffusion coefficient, and the water solubility of the gases involved. Oxygen, nitrous oxide, and carbon dioxide are soluble and move readily to establish equilibrium with a gas cavity. Nitrogen, sulfur hexafluoride, and perfluoropropane are insoluble. Therefore, they remain in the eye for prolonged periods and diffuse only slowly into solution to help reestablish equilibrium.

In a patient's eye, an insoluble gas bubble reaches equilibrium with the gases in the blood. When the patient is anesthetized with a mixture of 50% oxygen and 50% nitrous oxide, both of which are highly soluble gases, rapid expansion of the bubble occurs with oxygen and nitrous oxide diffusing into the cavity. The effect may also occur, but to a lesser extent, with 100% oxygen. Careful attention should be paid to the effect on intraocular pressure of anesthetic induction and the surgeon should be prepared to decompress the eye rapidly through the limbus or pars plana with a 30-gauge needle.

Once the patient is intubated and breathing a gas mixture of oxygen and nitrous oxide, attention must be paid to the effect of these mixtures on gas bubbles injected during surgery. If an air pump is used, the intraocular pressure is controlled by the pump. If air is moving through the eye, the mixture in the eye remains that of air. Once the eye is closed and movement of air ceases, oxygen and nitrous oxide start to diffuse into the eye. If equilibrium is established in the anesthetized state, the bubble will shrink when the patient awakens because the nitrous oxide and some of the oxygen will diffuse out of the eye. If the air is injected with a closed system, the bubble volume will expand rapidly while the patient breathes nitrous oxide and will become smaller when the patient breathes room air. The way to avoid these changes and their somewhat unpredictable effect is to have the patient breathe a mixture as close to air as is practical. If the patient is breathing nitrous oxide, it takes about 10 minutes to wash the nitrous oxide out of the system. Try to have the patient weaned from nitrous oxide for 10 minutes before closing the system.

Combined Technique

The idea of giving both local and general anesthetic might sound bizarre at first. After using the combined technique for many years, I enthusiastically support its use. Patients who are quite ill can tolerate the minimal anesthesia necessary for maintaining intubation. In this situation I do a subconjunctival injection as mentioned above and then follow with posterior irrigation of 0.5% bupivacaine (Marcaine). In all patients undergoing general anesthesia, I do posterior irrigation of bupivacaine (Marcaine) because of the excellent postoperative analgesia.

Minimal Anesthesia

Retinal surgery, particularly limited vitrectomies, can be done with a technique of topical drops followed by subconjunctival injection and posterior irrigation. Once the conjunctiva is opened, posterior irrigation using a blunt canula is carried out. I find this technique most useful for cooperative patients and limited surgery.

Summary

Any retinal procedures can be done with local anesthesia, but as the surgery becomes more complex, the advantages of general anesthesia outweigh the risks. The traditional Atkinson position of gaze and use of long (greater than $1^1/_4$ inch) needles should be abandoned. Sharp needles and slow injection make a retrobulbar injection tolerable for even the most pain-sensitive patients. A combined anesthetic of retrobulbar injection and general anesthesia is an excellent approach for dealing with sick patients who require long, complex retinal procedures.

Suggested Reading

Antoszyk AN, Buckley KG. Contralateral decreased visual acuity and extraocular muscle palsies following retrobulbar anesthesia. *Ophthalmology* 1986;93:462.

Fanning GL. Sedation techniques. *Ophthalmology Clinics of North America* 1998;11:73.

Gills JP, Hustead RF, Sanders DR. *Ophthalmic Anesthesia.* Thorofare, NJ: Slack Incorporated; 1993.

Javitt JC, Addiego R, Friedberg HL, et al. Brain stem anesthesia after retrobulbar block. *Ophthalmology* 1987;94:718.

Koornneef L. *Spatial Aspects of Orbital Musculo-Fibrous Tissue in Man.* Amsterdam: Swets & Zeitlinger; 1977.

Lincoff HE, Sweifach P, Brodie S, et al. Intraocular injection of lidocaine. *Ophthalmology* 1985;92:1587.

Linn JG, Smith BR. Intraoperative complications and their management. *Int Ophthalmol Clin* 1973;13(2):149.

Pautler SE, Grizzard WS, Thompson LN, Wing GL. Blindness from retrobulbar injection into the optic nerve. *Ophthalmic Surg* 1986;17:334.

Seelenfreund MH, Freilich DB. Retinal injuries associated with cataract surgery. *Am J Ophthalmol* 1980;89:654.

Sullivan KL, Brown GC, Forman AR, et al. Retrobulbar anesthesia and retinal vascular obstruction. *Ophthalmology* 1983;90:373.

Unsold R, Stanley JA, DeGroot I. The CT-topography of retrobulbar anesthesia. *Graefes Arch Clin Ophthalmol* 1981;217:137.

Wittpenn JR, Rapoza P, Sternberg P Jr, et al. Respiratory arrest following retrobulbar anesthesia. *Ophthalmology* 1986;93:867.

7

Scleral Buckling Surgery (Cryopexy and Explants)

Andrew J. Packer

Rhegmatogenous retinal detachments are caused by retinal breaks, usually resulting from vitreoretinal traction. The main goals of retinal reattachment surgery are to relieve the vitreoretinal traction and to close the retinal breaks (so that fluid from the vitreous cavity cannot gain access to the sub-retinal space). Once the retinal breaks are closed, remaining subretinal fluid will be removed by the retinal pigment epithelial "pump." In some instances of retinal detachment, vitreoretinal traction is minimal and retinal breaks can be treated with pneumatic retinopexy (see Chapter 5). At other times, severe vitreoretinal traction necessitates vitrectomy surgery (see Chapter 8).

Scleral buckling surgery accomplishes the goal of reattachment by indenting the underlying sclera, choroid, and retinal pigment epithelium with buckling elements (i.e., solid silicone tires or silicone sponges) to relieve mechanically the vitreoretinal traction and approximate the edges of the retinal break to the underlying retinal pigment epithelium. Buckling elements sutured to the external surface of the sclera are called *explants*, *exoplants*, or *episcleral implants*. If the sclera is dissected, the imbedded buckling material is called a *scleral implant*. The choroid and retinal pigment epithelium (RPE) in the vicinity of all of the retinal breaks is treated with a thermal irritant (i.e., cryopexy, diathermy, or laser photocoagulation) to form a permanent chorioretinal adhesion (i.e., a permanent seal) surrounding the retinal break. Frequently, it is necessary to drain subretinal fluid in order to close the retinal breaks. In this chapter, the surgical technique discussed is limited to explants and cryopexy. In general, this combination decreases operating time, minimizes complications, and allows easier intraoperative readjustment of the buckle, if necessary.

As mentioned in Chapter 2, a crucial part of the procedure is identifying all of the retinal breaks, since there are frequently more than one. The large, detailed fundus drawing should always be available in the operating room. Fundus landmarks in the drawing (such as vortex veins, retinal vessels, and regions of lattice degeneration) can help the surgeon to locate retinal breaks if intraoperative media problems prevent adequate visualization.

Preoperative Management

Once the decision is made to perform scleral buckling surgery, it is important that selected cases be performed in a timely manner. "Macula-on" and recent "macula-off" (i.e., up to 5 days) retinal detachments should be operated upon as soon as possible, preferably within 48 hours. Since outer segments of the retina depend upon blood supply from the choriocapillaris, prompt reattachment of the macula (or prevention of a macular detachment) maximizes the chance of preserving good vision. Chronic "macula-off" retinal detachments can be scheduled electively. Eyes with retinal detachments must be kept dilated (with atropine 1.0% or scopolamine 0.25%) between the time of diagnosis and the time of the operative procedure; failure to do so may result in iritis, miosis, and posterior synechiae, which may require additional surgery to visualize the fundus and reattach the retina.

The choice of general or local anesthesia is considered in detail in Chapter 6. If the surgeon (and patient) prefer general anesthesia, medical problems must be identified immediately so that medical consultation may be sought. Patients with hemoglobinopathies, particularly the sickle cell varieties, are at great risk for the development of anterior segment necrosis and this must be taken into account when surgical options are considered. The fundus drawings should ideally be performed, or at least rechecked, within 24–48 hours of surgery, since certain parameters (such as amounts of subretinal fluid or vitreous hemorrhage) may change over time.

Patients with "macula-on" retinal detachments threatening the macula are kept at bed rest until the surgery can be performed. Reading should be discouraged since saccadic eye movements can lead to further accumulation of subretinal fluid. Watching a distant television is not a problem since this requires little, if any, angular eye movements. Pinhole glasses also can limit extraocular movements. The patient's head should be positioned so that subretinal fluid remains away from the macula.

If elevated intraocular pressure is anticipated during surgery (i.e., large buckle required, little subretinal fluid to drain), patients may be treated with pressure lowering drops (i.e., beta blockers, or carbonic anhydrase inhibitors) or systemic acetazolamide preoperatively. Intravenous mannitol (1 g/kg) can also be used preoperatively or intraoperatively. Immediately prior to surgery (30–45 minutes), three sets of cyclopentolate 1.0% and phenylephrine 2.5% drops are administered at approximately 10-minute intervals. Topical antibiotic drops are also given. Since phenylephrine 10% is more likely to cause marked elevations in systemic blood pressure, its use, when necessary, is reserved for the operating room, where better patient monitoring is available. Care must of course be taken when dilating eyes with iris-fixated intraocular lenses.

Surgical Techniques

Opening

When positioning the patient's head (preferably on a donut-shaped pillow or a rolled towel), the chin should be elevated slightly, so that the brow and the lower orbital rim form a horizontal plane. The lid of the opposite eye is closed with tape if general anesthesia is used. If examination, cryopexy, or indirect laser photocoagulation is scheduled on the contralateral eye, dilating drops should be instilled in that eye to avoid delays at the conclusion of the scleral buckling surgery. The lids, brow, and upper cheek are scrubbed with a 10% povidone-iodine (Betadine) solution. Cotton-tipped applicators are used to cleanse the lashes. A drop of 5% povidone-iodine is placed in the conjunctival sac. The eye and lids are then rinsed with sterile water and the periorbital area is dried with a sterile towel. Alcohol can then be used to swab the lids.

A plastic adhesive drape with iodophor on the "sticky" side can be used as a further precaution against infection. A horizontal incision is made in the drape within the palpebral fissure unless a fenestrated drape is used. The conjunctiva (including the fornices) is then vigorously rinsed with a physiologic saline solution. Adequate exposure is usually provided with a lid speculum although on rare occasions, a lateral canthotomy is needed.

A 360-degree limbal peritomy is usually performed (unless a segmented buckle is anticipated). A radial cut is first made temporally by grasping a conjunctival fold near the limbus and cutting down on it adjacent to the limbus (Figure 7-1A). The conjunctiva (together with Tenon's capsule) is then undermined, using blunt Wescott scissors, and the incision made close to the limbus (Figure 7-1B). A more posterior peritomy can be performed in one or more quadrants if needed (for example, if a functioning filtration bleb is present). The conjunctiva must always be handled carefully, to prevent buttonholing, especially when it is thin and atrophic (as in elderly patients). At this point it is a good idea to check pupillary dilatation and add more topical drops if needed.

Tenon's space in the four quadrants is then carefully opened, with blunt dissection (using blunt, curved scissors, see Figure 7-2), attempting to avoid damage to the vortex veins. A cotton-tipped applicator is then used to strip the intermuscular fascia from the extraocular muscles. The four recti mus-

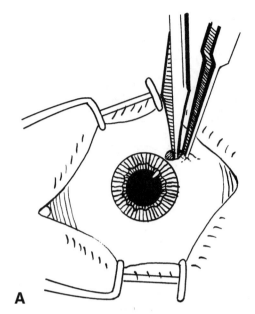
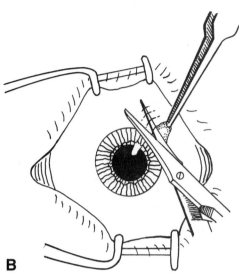

Figure 7-1. A, B, Limbal peritomy is performed.

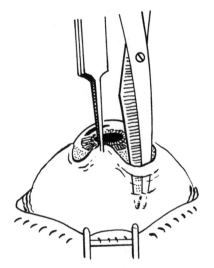

Figure 7-2. Blunt, curved scissors are used to open Tenon's space in the four quadrants.

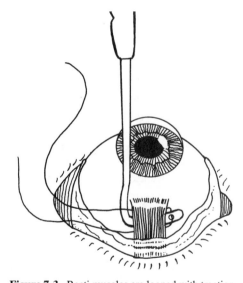

Figure 7-3. Recti muscles are looped with traction sutures.

cles are looped and traction sutures of 3-0 silk passed beneath their tendons with fenestrated muscle hooks (Figure 7-3). It is important to isolate the entire muscle tendon during this step and not "split" the muscle. The oblique muscles are purposely avoided (superiorly, the muscle hook should be passed from the superotemporal to the superonasal quadrant, to avoid the superior oblique). Knots are tied close to the muscle and at approximately 4

inches away; this helps to prevent tangling with buckle sutures later in the operation.

Muscle removal is virtually never required in scleral buckling surgery. If necessary, a double arm suture of 5-0 Vicryl with a spatula needle is passed through the ends of the muscle tendon close to the muscle insertion before the muscle is removed. Both needles are left on the long sutures for later reattachment to the sclera.

The scleral surface is then examined. This is best accomplished by grasping two adjacent traction sutures and pushing Tenon's capsule and conjunctive aside with a small retractor (Figure 7-4). This examination should document the occurrence of anomalous vortex veins, as well as regions of scleral thinning (scleral dehiscence) and staphyloma.

The surgeon must avoid damaging the cornea during the entire procedure, to optimize visualization of the fundus. The cornea is periodically moistened with physiologic saline solution or a 1–2% methylcellulose solution. The cornea may also be protected with a moistened Weck sponge. If the cornea becomes cloudy during the procedure, the epithelium can readily be removed with a No. 69 or No. 64 Beaver blade, or a No. 15 Bard-Parker blade by dragging the blade from the periphery toward the visual axis (Figure 7-5). It is important to avoid damaging Bowman's membrane during this maneuver. A rim of intact corneal epithelium (at least 1–2 mm) should be left in the periphery, if possible.

Localizing Retinal Breaks

Indirect ophthalmoscopy is used to locate the retinal breaks, usually with a 20-diopter lens. As previously mentioned, it is helpful to have the large fundus drawing available in the operating room at this time. A 28- or 30-diopter lens can be used if the pupil is small. The surgeon then performs scleral depression with a moistened, cotton-tipped applicator or instrument to localize the exact position of the retinal breaks on the corresponding external surface of the sclera. The straight (O'Conner) scleral

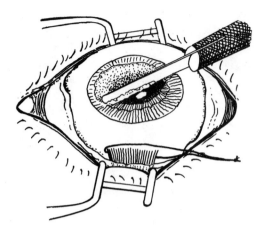

Figure 7-5. The corneal epithelium can be removed if it becomes cloudy.

marker is particularly helpful for posterior breaks (Figure 7-6). The assistant can help the surgeon by grasping two of the muscle sutures 180 degrees apart and rotating the eye so that the area of interest is directly opposite the surgeon.

If considerable scarring is present on the surface of the sclera, it can be difficult to identify a scleral mark. In this situation, a toothed forceps (0.3 mm) can be used to indent and then grasp the sclera at the appropriate location. The grasped area can then be marked.

If the retinal break is small, just the posterior margin need be marked. If it is large, the lateral margins should also be included. Large "horseshoe"

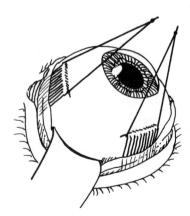

Figure 7-4. Retractors are used to examine the scleral surface.

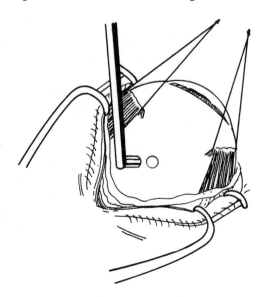

Figure 7-6. Retinal breaks are marked on the sclera.

tears usually require three marks to localize the posterior margin, as well as the extent of the two anterior horns (Figure 7-7). A sterile marking pen (felt-tipped) is used on the scleral surface and the ink "tatooed" with diathermy (or a disposable cautery). The localization should be checked; this can be readily accomplished by placing the back end of a cotton-tipped applicator on the scleral mark and depressing while viewing the fundus with the indirect ophthalmoscope.

Areas of lattice degeneration usually should be marked so that bands (or buckles) can cover the regions, particularly if retinal breaks are present and areas are treated with cryopexy.

After the retinal breaks are found, it is recommended that the surgeon examine the eye one final time by depressing the ora serrata 360 degrees in the hope of finding previously unrecognized retinal pathologic conditions. A wet, cotton-tipped applicator can be rolled continuously over the retinal periphery to ensure completeness of the examination.

Thermal Modalities

Cryopexy

Cryopexy should be performed to the regions surrounding each retinal break and to the areas of lattice degeneration. Contiguous freezes are applied, usually in a V-shape for horseshoe tears. Treatment is usually

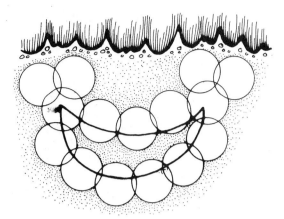

Figure 7-8. Cryopexy is placed around the margins of the large "horseshoe" tears.

extended to the ora serrata for anterior or equatorial tears. For large tears, one full row of freezes is placed peripheral to the margins of the retinal break (Figure 7-8). Treatment of bare RPE in the middle of large retinal breaks should be avoided since this serves no purpose and may cause dispersion of viable RPE cells into the vitreous cavity (leading to subsequent periretinal membrane formation).

If the cryoprobe is used to indent the outer eye wall, the RPE frequently can be brought into contact with the retina. In this situation, the endpoint of the treatment is the instant the first whitening appears within the retina (the foot pedal should be immediately released at this point to avoid overtreatment).

If the RPE cannot be brought into close proximity to the retina, a color change (pale yellow) frequently can be seen in the RPE itself; this represents an alternative endpoint. Freezing can take place relatively quickly in an eye with thin sclera and/or choroid (i.e., a myopic eye). Freezing also takes place rapidly in an air-filled eye (if the treated section of the retina is in contact with the air).

Care must be taken always to slide the cryoprobe under the conjunctive and rectus muscles and to direct the functioning portion of the probe against the scleral surface. The position of the opening of the protective plastic sheath covering the probe must always be checked. It is helpful to have an assistant call out temperature readings during the procedure. The endpoint should take place by approximately –40°C, if the sclera and choroid are of normal thickness. Freezes below –50°C usually

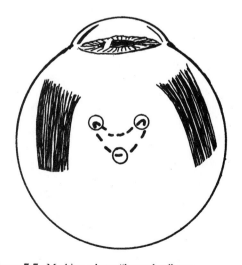

Figure 7-7. Marking a large "horseshoe" tear.

should be avoided. It is helpful to stop the procedure at such a point and check to be sure that the cryoprobe is indeed in contact with the scleral surface (and not on an extraocular muscle or lid). The surgeon must always be sure to view the tip of the probe and not the shaft, to avoid inadvertent posterior freezing that may affect the macula or the optic nerve; this is particularly true for straight probes (refer to Figure 4-1). As mentioned in Chapter 4, it is important to allow the probe to thaw completely (with the help of irrigating fluid) before separating it from the scleral surface to avoid the unnecessary risk of choroidal hemorrhage.

When the retina is highly elevated in the vicinity of a retinal break, it may be more accurate to mark or recheck the position of the retinal breaks after the cryopexy has been performed, since the latter frequently softens the eye and allows deeper scleral depression.

Laser

If any of the retinal breaks are present in areas of attached retina or in areas of shallow subretinal fluid, the indirect laser ophthalmoscope can be used to treat the retinal breaks. This can also be effective for treating flat areas of lattice if clinically indicated.

Transscleral diode laser probes have recently been used to treat retinal breaks during scleral buckling surgery though lack of widespread availability has limited its use. Transscleral diode lasers have the potential advantage of being able to function through existing silicone explants.

Choice of Explant

In general, the choice of explant in scleral buckling surgery is influenced by the following factors:

1. Size, number, and location of retinal breaks
2. Amount of vitreoretinal traction
3. Aphakia or pseudophakia
4. Available volume for the buckle (amount of subretinal fluid that can be safely drained)
5. Distribution of the subretinal fluid
6. Presence of proliferative vitreoretinopathy (PVR)
7. "Geography" of the scleral surface
8. Concern for choroidal detachment

Although the choice of the buckling hardware is always based upon the previous experience of the individual surgeon, it is beneficial for the retinal surgeon to be as open-minded as possible to alternative buckling techniques. This flexibility will allow for optimal results, particularly in challenging cases. The buckling element can either be circumferential (parallel to the limbus) or radial (perpendicular to the limbus). The two most widely used materials are solid silicone and silicone sponge. The solid silicone "tires" are usually grooved to accommodate an overlying band.

A wide variety of solid silicone bands, strips, tires, and accessories are available; several popular styles are illustrated in Figure 7-9. Commonly used varieties of silicone sponge explants are illustrated in Figure 7-10. Categories of explant configuration are shown in Figure 7-11.

As a general rule, during scleral buckling surgery all retinal breaks need to be covered by the

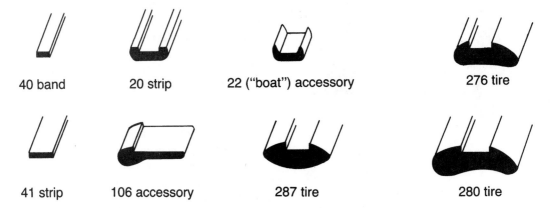

40 band	20 strip	22 ("boat") accessory	276 tire
41 strip	106 accessory	287 tire	280 tire

Figure 7-9. Commonly used solid silicone bands, strips, tires, and accessories.

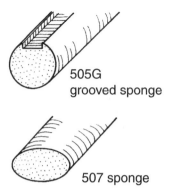
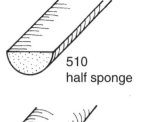
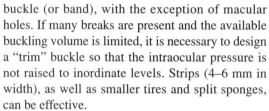
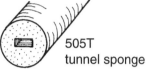

505G
grooved sponge

510
half sponge

507 sponge

505T
tunnel sponge

Figure 7-10. Examples of silicone sponge explants.

buckle (or band), with the exception of macular holes. If many breaks are present and the available buckling volume is limited, it is necessary to design a "trim" buckle so that the intraocular pressure is not raised to inordinate levels. Strips (4–6 mm in width), as well as smaller tires and split sponges, can be effective.

Encirclement (i.e., with either a band or a 360-degree circumferential buckle) is specifically recommended in the following circumstances:

1. Treatment of aphakic and pseudophakic retinal detachment
2. Multiple retinal breaks and/or large tears
3. No retinal break found
4. Preretinal membrane formation, star folds, vitreous membranes, PVR
5. High myopia
6. Extensive drainage of subretinal fluid
7. Extensive lattice degeneration
8. Desire to create a permanent buckling effect

It is frequently not necessary to drain subretinal fluid; it is however, necessary to close the retinal breaks. Buckle sutures can be temporarily tied to check for closure of retinal breaks without drainage. Drainage of subretinal fluid may also be necessary to allow for the volume displacement required for the buckling elements. In general, situations that tend to favor drainage include:

1. Longstanding retinal detachment (with viscous subretinal fluid that may require long periods of time for resorption)
2. Highly elevated retinal detachment (particularly with elevated retinal breaks)
3. Inferior retinal breaks
4. Presence of PVR

5. Absence of a recognized retinal break
6. Elderly patients (with poorly functioning RPE "pumps")
7. Eyes that cannot tolerate intraocular pressure elevations (i.e., recent intraocular surgery, severe glaucoma)

Radially oriented buckles are most effective for treating single, large, posterior horseshoe tears. This can prevent the posterior gaping of retinal tears ("fish-mouthing") that can result with circumferential buckles. In addition to freestanding radial sponges, radial accessories may be placed beneath circumferential buckles (see Figure 7-11B) to prevent the fish-mouthing.

Segmental circumferential buckles (usually of silicone sponge) can be used to treat straightforward anterior breaks, when the pathologic condition is limited to discrete regions (i.e., clock hours) and buckle height is not crucial. It also can be helpful if limited buckling volume is available.

As a general rule, solid silicone explants produce broader buckles and sponge explants produce higher indentation. For this reason, subretinal fluid need not be drained in a higher proportion of cases in which sponges are used.

When planning a circumferential solid silicone buckle, the following recommendations should be considered:

1. Bands or strips may be used to support small retinal breaks, as well as areas of lattice degeneration.
2. Extend the explant at least 15–30 degrees beyond the margins of the retinal break.
3. When possible, position the posterior margin of the retinal break near the middle of the tire width.

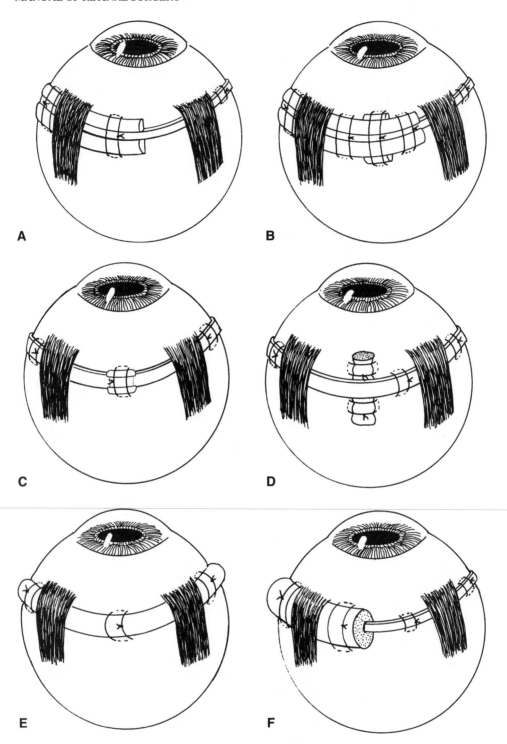

Figure 7-11. Categories of explant configuration. **A,** circumferential silicone tire with encircling band; **B,** circumferential silicone tire with underlying accessory; **C,** silicone strip with "boat" accessory; **D,** radial sponge with overlying encircling band; **E,** circumferential sponge; **F,** tunnel sponge with internally threaded encircling band.

4. Attempt to extend the buckle anteriorly to cover the ora serrata to prevent anterior leakage (an anterior "gutter"); see Figure 7-12. Suture placement at the line of muscle insertion will accomplish this goal. If the posterior extent of the planned tire is inadequate, an accessory can provide adequate posterior coverage, yet allow the anterior buckle suture to be placed near the muscle insertion line. The posterior suture should be placed at least 3-mm posterior to the posterior margin of the actual break.

Although it is desirable to place the circumferential buckle around the greater curvature of the eye (to prevent band migration), this can lead to vortex compression if the band is placed too far posteriorly. I find it best to keep the band between the equator and the ora serrata; this provides the best support for the ever-threatening vitreous base and minimizes vortex compression.

The following recommendations pertain to the use of radial sponges:

1. The diameter of the radial explant should be at least twice the width of the retinal break (i.e., if the retinal break is 2.5 mm across, a sponge at least 5 mm in diameter should be used).
2. Posterior coverage is crucial; start posterior radial sutures at the posterior margin of the retinal break and continue 2–3 mm posteriorly. If exposure is a problem, both suture bites may be made in the same anterior to posterior direction (Figure 7-13).

3. If the posterior extent of the radial sponge approaches the macula, use the "great toe" suture to avoid macular distortion (see following "Intrascleral Suture Placement" section).
4. Tie buckle sutures slowly (using temporary ties) to avoid excessive intraocular pressure elevation; watch the optic nerve head for arterial closure. (Paracentesis can be used to lower intraocular pressure; it is safest in phakic eyes or pseudophakic eyes with an intact posterior capsule.)
5. Trim radial sponges at the line of muscle insertion.
6. Close Tenon's capsule to the anterior muscle insertion (and episclera) in quadrants where radial sponges are used.

If a retinal break cannot be identified, it is a good idea to encircle the eye, supporting the vitreous base, since small, unrecognized breaks are most likely to be present in this location. Suspicious areas in the vicinity of the vitreous base are treated with cryopexy. Many surgeons prefer to drain subretinal fluid in this situation. As mentioned in Chapter 2, the location of retinal breaks can frequently be suspected by examining the distribution of the subretinal fluid. Suspected clock hours (for retinal breaks) should also be treated with two rows of cryopexy if a definite retinal break cannot be identified.

It is important to realize that most retinal breaks can be fixed with a variety of explant configurations.

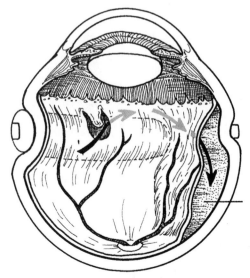

Figure 7-12. Anterior "gutter" can develop if buckle does not cover anterior portion of retinal break.

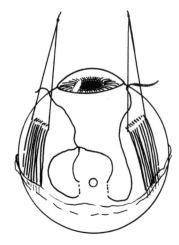

Figure 7-13. Posterior radial sutures placement for sponges should start at the posterior margin of the retinal break.

Geography of the scleral surface should be carefully examined before a course of action is chosen. For example, if a circumferential buckle is selected, yet would require suture placement through (or close to) a vortex vein, a radial sponge can be chosen instead. Similarly, a radial sponge may require a vertical suture through an area of thin sclera, and this may be better accomplished with horizontally placed sutures for a circumferential buckle, with or without an accessory.

Once the buckle configuration has been chosen, the appropriate explant material should be soaked in an antibiotic solution.

Intrascleral Suture Placement

For circumferential buckles, one to two buckle sutures are usually placed in each quadrant, preferably directly over the retinal breaks. In general, explant segments should be secured by at least two buckle sutures. Suture material should be of the permanent variety. Nylon has the advantage of allowing the surgeon to tie the sutures without assistance (with a three-one-one tie). Colored sutures may be easier to find if reoperation is subsequently required. Suture needles should be of the spatula type (quarter or half circle). Half-circle needles are particularly helpful for posterior suture placement.

The sclera is engaged with the tip of the needle to approximately half depth and the needle is then passed along the same plane for a total length of 2–3 mm (Figure 7-14). Other surgeons prefer longer scleral bites (as long as 5 mm). Since suture placement is difficult in soft eyes, it is helpful to raise the intraocular pressure in such eyes by placing cotton-tipped applicators adjacent to the globe 180 degrees away.

Fixation of a rectus tendon with a toothed forceps for countertraction is helpful for suture placement. Bluish-appearing areas of sclera represent thin regions and should be avoided.

Sutures are placed in a mattress fashion, according to the orientation of the buckling element. The free ends of the suture are held together with a Serrefine clamp until the sutures are tied.

The distance between the anterior and posterior bites for silicone tires should be approximately 2 mm larger than the actual width of the explant. The appropriate distance is usually printed on the explant's packaging label. The use of accessories

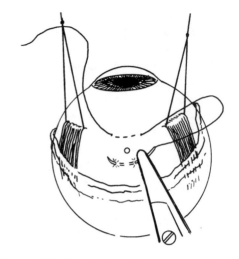

Figure 7-14. Intrascleral buckle sutures are placed with the needle at approximately half depth.

requires modification (for example, the suggested width for a No. 276 tire with underlying No. 106 button is 13 mm). Buckle height can be enhanced by wider suture placement.

If a sponge explant is used, the distance between the suture bites should be 1.5 times the diameter of the sponge.

Radial sponges can produce a "dimpling" effect that extends posteriorly from the margin of the sponge. "Toe sutures" can be used to avoid potential macular distortion. As shown in Figure 7-15A, the ends of the regularly placed posterior vertical mattress suture are left long and an additional scleral bite is taken at the posterior margin of the sponge; in Figure 7-15B, the ends are tied, which limits the posterior dimpling effect of the sponge.

If the suture is placed too deeply (penetrating the sclera, choroid, pigment epithelium, and possibly retina) and/or fluid is noted to leak from the needle tract, the tract should usually be marked and the suture removed and placed more posteriorly. The underlying retina is then examined with indirect ophthalmoscopy and, if a retinal break is noted, it is treated accordingly. The indirect laser can be useful in this situation if the retina is attached; cryopexy can also be used. Continued drainage of liquid vitreous or subretinal fluid may be stopped with shallow scleral sutures of 7-0 Vicryl, although this is rarely necessary.

Band sutures are placed in a very shallow fashion, to avoid unnecessary risk of scleral perforation. The

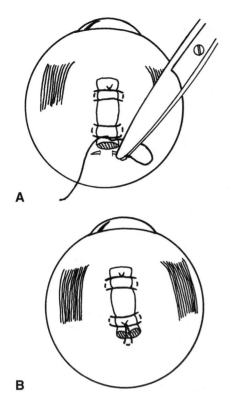

A

B

Figure 7-15. A, B, "Toe sutures" can avoid potential macular distortion.

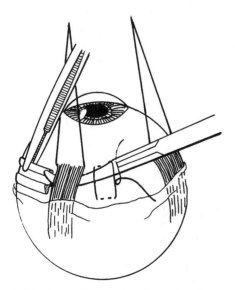

Figure 7-16. A curved hemostat can be used to place circumferential buckling elements beneath sutures and muscles.

anterior and posterior bites are placed approximately 3 mm apart for a 2-mm band. One band suture is placed in each quadrant that does not already contain at least one buckle suture. When all sutures have been placed, buckling elements are positioned appropriately beneath the sutures and the recti muscles. Grooved, circumferential explants with the overlying bands are grasped together by a small, curved hemostat that has been placed beneath the buckle sutures and muscles (Figure 7-16).

Drainage of Subretinal Fluid

As previously mentioned, subretinal fluid need be drained only when retinal breaks cannot otherwise be closed. Buckle sutures can be temporarily tied to check for closure of the retinal breaks without drainage.

In general, it is desirable to drain subretinal fluid:

1. Away from the retinal breaks (particularly large breaks) to prevent drainage of liquid vitreous through the retinal breaks
2. Beneath the areas of maximal retinal elevation
3. Beneath retinal star folds (since these areas of the retina tend to remain elevated until other areas of the retina flatten)
4. In the bed of the buckle (under preplaced buckle sutures)

Areas adjacent to the lateral rectus muscle are the most desirable because of the easy accessibility. It is important to avoid areas adjacent to vortex veins (i.e., mid-quadrant), because of the higher risk of choroidal bleeding. Anterior drainage sites are preferable, again, to limit the risk of choroidal bleeding. It is prudent to recheck the configuration of the subretinal fluid immediately before drainage, since the subretinal fluid may shift when the eye position is altered and buckling elements are positioned.

The drainage site is prepared by radially oriented cuts in the sclera with a No. 64 or No. 69 Beaver blade. Diathermy to the scleral lips (using a conical tip) can be used to open the scleral wound by lateral tissue contraction. The endpoint of the scleral dissection (3–4 mm in length) is the herniation of a small, dark knuckle of choroid into the lips of the scleral wound (Figure 7-17A). If bleeding is noted from the choroidal surface or if large choroidal vessels are seen, the site is abandoned and a new one chosen.

The choroidal surface can be readily examined with loupes or with the magnification of a 20-diopter lens using the indirect ophthalmoscope. A preplaced suture (of nylon) is placed in the lips of the scleral incision if the drain site is not in the bed of the buckle (Figure 7-17B). The scleral lips are then held open with a fine-toothed forceps (0.12 mm) and all traction is released on the globe. If the intraocular pressure is still elevated, some of the preplaced buckling material must be temporarily removed to normalize the intraocular pressure prior to drainage.

I favor light diathermy to the choroidal bed as a precaution against choroidal bleeding, prior to penetration of the choroid and pigment epithelium with a sharp suture needle (see Figure 7-17B). Alternatively, a diathermy pin or 30-gauge needle (with a 90-degree bend) can be used. Penetration is promptly stopped and the needle withdrawn when fluid leakage is first noted. Choroidal penetration can also be performed with a disposable cautery or with an argon endolaser probe. The latter technique is particularly useful if the retina is shallowly detached at the planned drainage site.

After choroidal penetration, fluid can be gently expressed using cotton-tipped applicators. The cotton-tipped applicators are placed adjacent to the globe to take up volume temporarily and prevent hypotony. It is desirable to place the drainage site in a gravitationally dependent position. Endpoints of drainage include stoppage of fluid flow, appearance of pigment, or appearance of blood. If stoppage of flow is followed by a sudden gush of fluid, retinal incarceration and perforation in the drainage

site must be suspected. The overlying buckle sutures (or intrascleral mattress sutures if the drain is not in the bed of the buckle) are then tied temporarily with slip knots and the retina examined with indirect ophthalmoscopy. One observes the amount of remaining subretinal fluid and its proximity to the drainage site, and looks carefully for possible complications, such as subretinal hemorrhage, retinal breaks at the drainage site, and retinal incarceration (which should be treated as would a retinal break). Again, the indirect laser ophthalmoscope can be particularly helpful in treating these breaks. Scleral depression is used on the buckle and one or two rows of laser are placed around the retinal break or incarceration.

If more fluid needs to be drained, the original drain site may be reopened (if it appears safe to do so) or a new drainage site selected. The original drainage site should never be reopened if hemorrhage is observed at the site. If subretinal hemorrhage is seen, the head should be positioned to avoid collection of the blood in the macula. This, of course, is not a concern with macula-on detachments.

An alternative technique for draining subretinal fluid can be performed using indirect ophthalmoscopy and a 25-gauge, $^5/_8$-inch needle attached to either a small syringe (without a plunger) or to the foot pedal-controlled linear suction of a vitrectomy system. The needle is advanced obliquely through the sclera (to allow self closure) avoiding larger choroidal vessels; the bevel of the needle is turned toward the RPE (to avoid retinal incarceration). Proponents of this technique prefer the con-

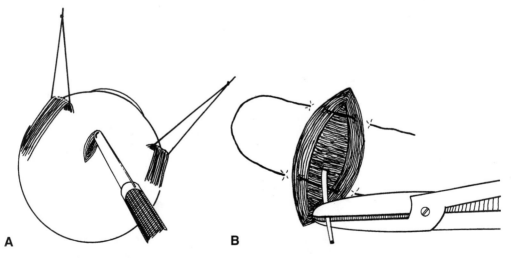

Figure 7-17. A, preparation of drainage site; **B,** penetration of choroid with a sharp needle.

trolled fluid egress and the simultaneous "internal" visualization.

When the drainage is completed, buckle sutures are pulled up and tied permanently. If a band is used, the ends may be joined with a permanent suture clove hitch or a Watzke sleeve. The ends of the encircling sponges (or tires) may be joined directly (end-to-end), using a permanent mattress suture.

While you are tying the buckle sutures, the intraocular pressure should be checked periodically. If it is elevated, the perfusion of the retinal arterioles (i.e., arterial pulsation near the optic nerve head) must be checked; the arterioles should be open at least 50% of the time. A paracentesis can be performed if the intraocular pressure is excessively high. This maneuver is safer in phakic eyes or pseudophakic eyes with an intact posterior capsule. A 30-gauge needle is introduced over the peripheral iris (to avoid risking damage to the lens) and approximately 0.1 ml of fluid withdrawn. A paracentesis knife can similarly be used. Paracentesis should be avoided in aphakic eyes because vitreous can be pulled to the limbal puncture site. I prefer to avoid removal of "liquid vitreous" via a pars plana needle, since formed vitreous can be withdrawn, causing increased vitreoretinal traction.

If pressure elevation is anticipated, temporary ties can be used and the tension loosened appropriately. Slow, intermittent tying of the buckle sutures is frequently an effective technique for dealing with elevated intraocular pressure. As previously mentioned, mannitol may be administered intravenously (1 g/kg) for marked intraocular pressure elevation.

After the subretinal fluid is drained, fundus visualization may be poor; this usually results from either a hazy cornea or a small pupil. Miosis may be corrected by topical drops in some instances. Epinephrine (0.1 ml of 1:10,000 concentration) can also be injected into the anterior chamber and argon endolaser photomydriasis used in refractory cases. Flexible iris retractors can be used in aphakic and pseudophakic eyes if visualization is crucial. Redirecting the light of the indirect ophthalmoscope upward and using a 28- or 30-diopter lens can also help to see through a small pupil. If the corneal epithelium appears edematous, it can sometimes be temporarily cleared by rolling a wet and squeezed-out cotton-tipped applicator over the corneal surface; the cornea is irrigated after the maneuver is completed and the fundus viewed promptly. It may also be necessary at this point to remove edematous corneal epithelium with a blade (as previously described).

The fundus is then reexamined to check the position of retinal breaks on the buckle. Although the margins of the retinal breaks need not be flat on the buckle, the buckle element must entirely underlie the retinal break. Indentation of the buckling element (with external pressure) may aid in this evaluation. If the retinal breaks are not sufficiently covered, buckle sutures may be repositioned or accessories placed with new buckle sutures. Figure 7-18 demonstrates the placement of a segment of circumferential sponge to the posterior margin of an existing explant for further posterior coverage; new sutures are placed to include both explants. If a radial sponge appears to be too narrow, new buckle sutures may be placed lateral to the existing sutures and a wider sponge used after the original is removed.

Physiologic saline solution, air, or expansile gases may be used to reconstitute the vitreous cavity after buckle sutures have been tied if the eye is hypotonus (though this is usually not necessary). Injections are made through the pars plana (measured 4 mm posterior to the limbus in phakic eyes and 3 mm posterior to the limbus in pseudophakic eyes) using a 30-gauge needle. In aphakic eyes (without a posterior capsule), the injection may be given through the limbus. In general, physiologic

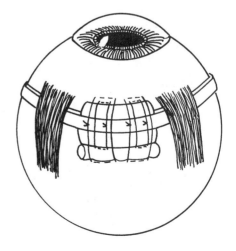

Figure 7-18. Placement of circumferential sponge along posterior margin of an existing explant.

saline is used when the retinal breaks are flat on the buckle. Air or expansile gas injections are used when an intraocular tamponade is required to close an elevated retinal break over a well-positioned buckle, or if "fish-mouthing" (posterior gaping of the tear) occurs. Air/gas bubbles are most effective when the breaks are located in the superior 8 hours, since inferior positioning of the bubble is difficult postoperatively.

Air/gas should always pass through a Millipore filter prior to intraocular injection. If the surgery is performed under general anesthesia, the anesthetist should be alerted to discontinue the nitrous oxide when air or gas bubbles are used, since nitrous oxide can drastically change the volume of the bubble in a very short time. If an expansile gas is used, topical beta blockers and carbonic anhydrase inhibitors should be administered postoperatively.

Concluding Surgery

The buckling elements and the subconjunctival space are irrigated with an antibiotic solution. Tenon's capsule should be attached to the anterior muscle insertion or episclera with 7-0 Vicryl sutures in quadrants where sponge material has been used (especially radially oriented sponges). This special two-layer closure helps to prevent sponge extrusion and infection.

The conjunctiva is closed with winged sutures of 7-0 Vicryl, incorporating episcleral tissue. Relaxing incisions and other dehiscences in the conjunctiva should be meticulously repaired to prevent buckle exposure, infection, and extrusion.

I prefer to inject subconjunctival cefazolin (20 mg), as well as peribulbar steroid (Kenalog, 40 mg) at the conclusion of the procedure. Atropine 1% drops (or ointment) and a combination antibiotic/steroid

ointment are also used. If the intraocular pressure is elevated, drops of timolol (0.5%) and topical carbonic anhydrase inhibitors may be used; acetazolamide (500 mg) may also be administered intravenously. As mentioned previously, pressure-lowering drops are always used when an expansile gas bubble is injected, and systemic acetazolamide is frequently used during the first 24 hours. The eye is then patched and a protective Fox shield is taped into place.

A detailed operative report is particularly helpful if postoperative problems are encountered and reoperation is required. A detailed diagram should be placed in the patient's chart that shows the location and types of buckling material used, as well as the locations of the drain sites.

Suggested Reading

Aaberg TM, Wiznia RA. The use of solid soft silicone rubber exoplants in retinal detachment surgery. *Ophthal Surg* 1976;7:98.

Charles ST. Controlled drainage of subretinal and choroidal fluid. *Retina* 1985;5:233–234.

Haller JA, Lim JI, Goldberg MF. Pilot trial of transscleral diode laser retinopexy in retinal detachment surgery. *Arch Ophthalmol* 1993;111:952.

Harris M, Blumenkrantz M, Wittpenn J, et al. Geometric alterations produced by encircling scleral buckles. *Retina* 1987;7:14.

Michels RG. Scleral buckling methods for rhegmatogenous retinal detachment. *Retina* 1986;6:1.

Regillo CD, Benson WE. *Retinal Detachment: Diagnosis and Management*. 3rd ed. Philadelphia: Lippincott-Raven; 1998:100–134.

Wilkenson CP, Rice TA. *Michels Retinal Detachment*. 2nd ed. Philadelphia: Mosby; 1997:537–594.

Williams GA, Aaberg TM. Techniques of scleral buckling. In: Ryan SJ, et al., eds. *Retina*. 2nd ed. St. Louis, MO: Mosby; 1994:1979–2017.

8

Posterior Segment Vitrectomy

Gary W. Abrams and Jane C. Werner

Goals of Vitrectomy

The term *vitrectomy* literally means to excise the vitreous. The vitrectomy operation, however, encompasses a wide range of surgical procedures within the posterior segment of the eye. In this chapter we will discuss the goals of and indications for vitrectomy and the instrumentation for vitrectomy procedures. We will describe the various components of a vitrectomy operation.

The major goals of a vitrectomy operation are listed in Table 8-1. A single vitrectomy procedure may have multiple goals.

Indications for Vitrectomy

The major indications for vitrectomy are listed in Table 8-2. Nonresolving vitreous opacities are of four basic types: hemorrhagic, inflammatory, metabolic, and neoplastic. Hemorrhage may result from diabetic or other proliferative retinopathies, retinal

Table 8-1. Major Goals of Vitrectomy

- Clear the media
- Relieve vitreoretinal traction
- Internal treatment of retinal breaks and retinal detachment
- Diagnosis
- Treat infection
- Remove foreign or unwanted material from the eye
- Treat macular disorders

tears, trauma, intraocular surgery, subarachnoid hemorrhage, avulsed retinal vessels, ocular tumors, and disciform processes. Inflammatory debris may result from various types of uveitides. The most common metabolic vitreous opacity is primary systemic or localized ocular amyloidosis. Large cell lymphoma is the most common cause of neoplastic vitreous opacification.

The most common proliferative retinopathy is diabetic retinopathy. Other proliferative retinopathies sometimes treated with vitrectomy are branch or central retinal vein occlusion, sickle cell retinopathy, Eales's disease, and other forms of vasculitis and obstructive retinopathies. Surgical indications for the proliferative retinopathies are usually long-standing vitreous hemorrhage and/or retinal detachment.

Vitrectomy may be indicated for complicated retinal detachments. A retinal detachment associated with vitreous hemorrhage may require vitrectomy prior to a scleral buckling procedure to allow the surgeon to visualize the retinal breaks. Some retinal detachments due to posterior retinal breaks are best treated with vitrectomy. Retinal detachment with proliferative vitreoretinopathy requires vitrectomy in its advanced stages to remove tractional membranes. Giant retinal tears may require vitrectomy in order to unfold the retina and introduce a tamponade (such as gas or silicone oil).

Macular epiretinal membranes may be idiopathic or follow retinal detachment surgery, cryopexy, laser photocoagulation, or be associated with various vascular retinopathies. Surgery is

Table 8-2. Indications for Vitrectomy

- Nonresolving vitreous opacities
- Proliferative retinopathies
- Traction retinal detachments
- Complicated rhegmatogenous retinal detachments
  - Retinal detachment with vitreous hemorrhage
  - Proliferative vitreoretinopathy
  - Posterior tears
  - Giant tears
  - Combined tractional-rhegmatogenous retinal detachments
- Posteriorly dislocated crystalline lens or lens material
- Posteriorly dislocated pseudophakos
- Epiretinal membranes, vitreomacular traction, and vitreopapillary traction
- Macular holes
- Subretinal neovascular membranes and/or subretinal hemorrhage
- Diagnostic vitrectomy
- Ocular trauma including intraocular foreign bodies
- Endophthalmitis
- Retinal detachment associated with retinopathy of prematurity
- Intravitreal ganciclovir implantation
- Other: uveitis and aphakic cystoid macular edema
- Foveal translocation

seldom indicated until the visual acuity is reduced to 20/60 or worse.

The whole lens or part of a lens may dislocate posteriorly during cataract surgery and may cause uveitis, glaucoma, or lead to retinal detachment. A dislocated lens may be secondary to Marfan's syndrome, homocystinuria, trauma, or syphilis. Posteriorly dislocated lenses are best managed with vitrectomy techniques.

A posteriorly dislocated pseudophakos may lead to posterior segment complications. By using vitrectomy techniques, a dislocated intraocular lens (IOL) can be either repositioned or removed.

Vitrectomy may be indicated to obtain a vitreous specimen for cytologic diagnosis of a neoplasm such as large cell lymphoma. Cultures can be obtained in suspected cases of endophthalmitis and a cellular diagnosis obtained in cases of uveitis. Vitrectomy for molecular diagnosis of several infectious organisms is now possible. In particular, PCR is useful for diagnosis of herpes viruses. In some centers, PCR diagnosis of syphilis, toxoplasmosis, bacteria, and fungi is available. Vitrectomy may also be indicated in uveitis to clear the media, to

treat tractional complications, and to remove cyclitic membranes.

Vitrectomy may be indicated in patients with aphakic or pseudophakic cystoid macular edema (CME) if vitreous is incarcerated in the wound or perhaps adherent to anterior intraocular structures. Vitrectomy for CME is controversial in eyes without vitreous incarceration.

In cases of endophthalmitis, vitrectomy is useful for obtaining a specimen for culture, as well as for removing inflammatory debris from the eye. In association with the use of intraocular antibiotics, the treatment of endophthalmitis has been greatly enhanced by vitrectomy techniques. Vitrectomy has been proven beneficial in the most advanced forms of endophthalmitis by the Endophthalmitis Vitrectomy Study.

Ocular trauma associated with penetrating injuries or intraocular foreign bodies is often managed with vitrectomy techniques. Penetrating injuries with severe hemorrhage with or without retinal detachment often require vitrectomy. Intraocular foreign bodies that are nonmagnetic, obscured by hemorrhage, incarcerated in tissue, or encapsulated usually require treatment with vitrectomy.

Retinopathy of prematurity in advanced stages may require vitrectomy. Newer lens-sparing vitrectomy techniques may improve visual rehabilitation following surgery in neonates, and the use of smaller, 25-gauge instruments should allow safer and more precise surgical maneuvers.

While not always requiring a vitrectomy, the use of ganciclovir implants has improved the quality of life of many patients by allowing them to stop or reduce the need for frequent intravenous or intravitreal antiviral therapy.

More recent indications for vitrectomy are for treatment of macular disorders such as macular hole, subretinal hemorrhage, and subfoveal neovascular membranes. Treatment of a macular hole requires vitrectomy, separation of the posterior cortical vitreous over the macula, dissection of epiretinal membranes, and possibly internal limiting membranes, and tamponade with a gas bubble. Subfoveal neovascular membranes and subretinal hemorrhages may be removed through small retinotomies following vitrectomy. The indications for the latter procedures are the subject of an ongoing national randomized clinical trial (Subretinal Surgery Trial) sponsored by the National Eye Institute. Foveal translocation techniques may offer the possibility of visual improvement for some patients with subfoveal choroidal neovascular membranes. Indications for these procedures have yet to be completely defined and randomized; controlled clinical trials are pending.

Instrumentation

Early vitreous cutting instruments were "full-function" instruments that provided cutting capability, suction, fluid infusion, and illumination in a single large probe. The full-function instrument was placed through a single large sclerotomy site. Modern instruments are of a "split-function" design, in which suction and cutting, infusion, and illumination are separated and placed through three individual small ports. By separating the function of the instruments, it was possible to reduce their size. The advantages of miniaturizing the instruments outweigh the disadvantages of the multiport system. Early instruments had a rotating or oscillating inner cutting tip, but most recent instruments use a "guillotine" cutting action. The guillotine cutting instrument (Figure 8-1) has an outer fixed tube (Figure 8-1A) with an opening (Figure 8-1B) through which vitreous is aspirated. An inner cutting tip (Figure 8-1C) slides across the inner portion of the opening to cut the vitreous. There is less risk of incarcerating vitreous in the opening of an instrument with a guillotine-type action than one with a rotating or oscillating action. Most instruments cut at a maximum of approximately 600 cycles per second. Some newer instruments have cutting rates of up to 1500 cycles per second that cause less traction on the retina when cutting unseparated vitreous such as at the vitreous base. Smaller diameter cutters, as small as 25 gauge, have been developed for use in small eyes.

Other instruments necessary for vitreous surgery are listed in Table 8-3. It is often difficult to predict which instruments will be necessary during an individual case, so we recommend that all instruments be available for most cases.

Table 8-3. Accessory Vitrectomy Instruments

- Microvitreoretinal blades (19 and 20 gauge)
- Scleral plugs and forceps
- Lens system
  - Hand-held infusion lenses
  - Sew-on lens ring set
    - Lenses for posterior pole, wide angle, peripheral viewing and fluid-gas exchange
  - Wide-angle system (contact vs. noncontact)
- Illumination system
  - Light source
  - Fiberoptic illumination probes
    - Standard
    - Wide-angle
    - Illuminated picks (Figure 8-2), knives, or forceps
- Ultrasound lens fragmentation unit
- Bipolar diathermy
  - Exodiathermy
  - Unimanual, bipolar endodiathermy
- Vitreoretinal picks
  - Barbed MVR blade
  - Michels picks
  - Illuminated picks
- Vitreous scissors
  - Right angle vertically cutting (Figure 8-3A)
  - Horizontally cutting (Figure 8-3B)
  - Automated handpiece
  - Membrane PeelerCutter (MPC) (Figure 8-4)
- Vitreous forceps
  - End-grabbing membrane
    - Various sizes and configurations
    - Diamond dusted (Figure 8-5A)
  - Machemer diamond dusted foreign body forceps (Figure 8-5B)
  - Subretinal forceps (Figure 8-5C)
  - Illuminated forceps
- Suction needles
  - Silicone-tipped
- Charles (fluted) needle and handle (backflush system preferred)
  - Backflush brush
  - Cannulated extrusion needle system (snake)
- Laser endophotocoagulation system
- Laser Indirect Ophthalmoscope
- Continuous infusion air-pump system
- Cryosurgical unit
- Perfluoropropane and SF_6 gases
- Silicone oil
- Perfluorocarbon liquid
- Tissue manipulator (Figure 8-6)
- Iris retractors
- Diamond-dusted membrane scraper
- Intraocular foreign body magnet

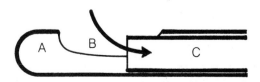

Figure 8-1. "Guillotine" vitreous cutter. Inner cylindrical blade (**C**) slides across opening (**B**) within outer tube (**A**).

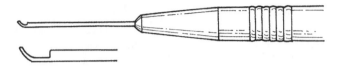

Figure 8-2. Fiberoptic illuminated pick.

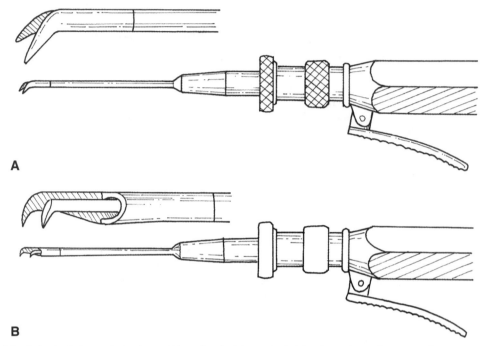

A

B

Figure 8-3. Sutherland vitreoretinal scissors (Alcon Surgical, Fort Worth, TX). **A,** Horizontally-cutting. **B,** Vertically-cutting.

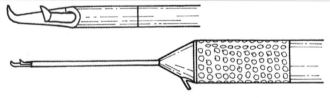

Figure 8-4. MPC vitreoretinal scissor (Alcon Surgical, Fort Worth, TX).

Preoperative Management

Ocular Examination

A complete general eye examination should be performed on both eyes of all patients prior to vitreous surgery (see Chapter 2). If the patient cannot read the Snellen chart, lower levels of visual acuity should be documented.

Of particular interest to the vitrectomy surgeon is the study of vitreoretinal relationships with slit-lamp biomicroscopy (i.e., using a Goldmann three-mirror or a 78- or 90-diopter noncontact aspheric lens). Cross-sectional vitreoretinal drawings can be most helpful in understanding complex vitreoretinal pathologic changes. Retinal drawings should include the degree of posterior vitreous separation and the areas of vitreo-retinal adhesion. Proliferative membranes and active neovascularization should be documented and areas of choroidal detachment and anterior cyclitic membrane (distorting the peripheral retina), which might interfere with instrument placement, should be noted.

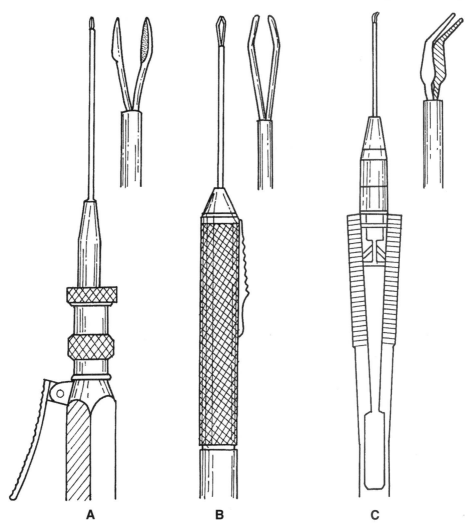

Figure 8-5. Vitreoretinal forceps. **A,** Sutherland diamond-dusted end-grabbing forcep (Alcon Surgical, Fort Worth, TX). **B,** Machemer diamond-dusted foreign body forcep (Alcon Surgical, Fort Worth, TX). **C,** Subretinal forcep (Synergetics, St. Louis, MO).

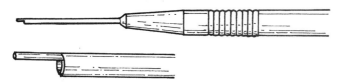

Figure 8-6. Tissue manipulator.

Corneal clarity must be carefully evaluated, since severe opacification might require the use of a temporary keratoprosthesis device. A donor cornea should be available at the time of surgery if the temporary keratoprosthesis is to be used.

As mentioned in Chapter 2, the iris should be meticulously examined prior to instillation of mydriatics to search for iris neovascularization (rubeosis iridis). Preoperative iris neovascularization is a particularly poor prognostic factor in diabetics, although prompt reattachment of a detached retina and extensive intraoperative endophotocoagulation may salvage the eye.

The lens should be carefully evaluated to determine both the clarity of the lens and the estimated "hardness" of the lens nucleus. It is usually easier to remove the lens early in the procedure; therefore, the decision to remove the lens is often made preoperatively. If an extremely hard lens nucleus is anticipated, the decision to perform a limbal extraction is sometimes made.

Surgical Planning

The surgeon should have a plan for the operation. Although findings and events at surgery may change the surgical design, careful preoperative planning will reduce the likelihood of intraoperative problems. The surgeon should anticipate the equipment needed for the procedure. Ultrasound lens fragmentation, scissors, forceps, or other equipment should be available as required (see Table 8-3). The surgeon should try to anticipate potential surgical complications.

Prior to induction of anesthesia, the operating microscope, the vitrectomy instrument and console, all foot pedals, and other critical instruments are checked for proper function. All equipment needed for the procedure should be available (see Table 8-3).

Anesthesia

Vitreous surgery can be performed under either local or general anesthesia (see Chapter 6). We use local anesthesia with close monitoring of the patient's medical condition by an anesthesiologist for most cases. We use general anesthesia for children and for adults unable to tolerate a local anesthetic. Examples of adults that might benefit from a general anesthetic include patients that are mentally challenged, highly anxious, or claustrophobic.

For local anesthesia, we require anesthesia standby with constant monitoring of the patient. We prefer a 50:50 mixture of 2% lidocaine (Xylocaine) and 0.75% bupivacaine as the local anesthetic agent. A lid block is usually not used. We give an injection of 5 ml of the anesthetic solution in the retrobulbar space. The patient may be placed on an air mattress for comfort. We create a tent over the patient's nose and mouth by elevating the drapes with a small cardboard device that adheres to the face with a Nevyas disposable drape retractor (Varitronics, Inc., Broomall, PA). Oxygen is delivered to the patient through a nasal catheter. High levels of oxygen should usually be avoided since this can promote retinal phototoxicity. Sedation may be beneficial for some patients, but it is important that the sedative be carefully titrated by an anesthesiologist experienced in local anesthesia. Patients should not be overly sedated because they may move upon awakening during the procedure.

Patient Preparation

We cleanse the skin and the eyelids with 10% povidone-iodine (Betadine) solution. We place 5% povidone-iodine in the conjunctival cul-de-sac. The head is centered on the headrest, leveled, and the face is directed toward the ceiling. Proper draping is critical to ensure a sterile, dry field and to protect personnel and equipment from fluids on the floor (Figure 8-7). We drape the forehead, then place a large plastic drape over the eye, draping out the eyelids, with an adhesive portion covering the eyelid and periocular skin. The nonadhesive portion of the drape covers the remainder of the face and the operative field. Figure 8-7 shows the draped patient and the trough around the head created in the drape between the head and the U-shaped wrist rest surrounding the top and sides of the head. Fluid is caught in the trough and is removed with a suction catheter.

Instrument Arrangement

A host of large instrument consoles and foot pedals are necessary for vitreous surgery. The instruments should be arranged in a convenient and safe manner that allows easy access to the patient by the operating room personnel. Foot pedals should be placed so that the surgeon can easily engage them while maintaining his or her balance. Consoles can be conveniently stacked on a neurosurgical table placed across and above the inferior portion of the operating table (Figure 8-8). A sterile plastic drape can be placed over the consoles.

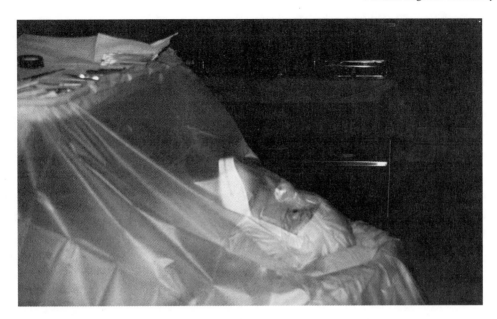

Figure 8-7. Patient draped for vitreoretinal surgery.

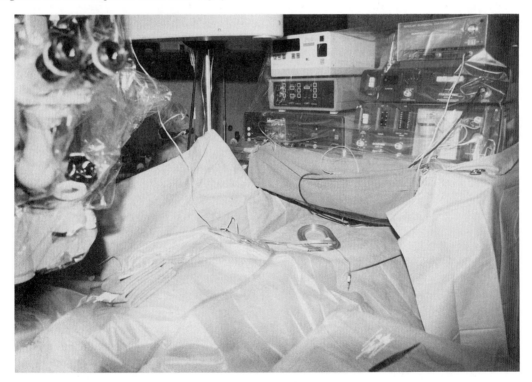

Figure 8-8. Instrument consoles stacked on neurosurgical table.

Intraocular Infusion Solutions

The intraocular solution for infusion should be sterile and isotonic, with constituents near those of normal ocular fluids and with a balanced pH. The following combination appears to be the best available ocular irrigating solution: (1) glutathione, which protects the cellular enzymes from oxidizing agents and is essential for maintaining intercellular junctions; (2) glucose, an energy source; (3) magnesium, an important factor in cellular enzymes; (4) a bicarbonate buffer system; and (5) Ringer's lactate solution. We use commercially available balanced salt solution (BSS plus, Alcon Laboratories, Fort Worth) for vitreous surgery.

Diabetic lenses may develop posterior subcapsular feathery opacities during vitrectomy due to excessive accumulation of glucose, fructose, and sorbitol, which induce osmotic uptake of water. We add 3 cc of 50% dextrose (without preservatives or antioxidants) to 500 cc BSS plus solution (which increases the glucose concentration to 400 mg/dl and increases the osmolality of the solution to 320 mOsm) to prevent lens opacification during diabetic vitrectomy. We use glucose-fortified BSS plus for diabetic patients and regular BSS plus (without additional glucose) for nondiabetic patients.

Preparation for Entrance into the Eye

Prior to entering the eye, we inspect and test the vitrectomy instrument and flush air bubbles from the system. We inspect the infusion port and run fluid through the tubing to flush out any remaining air. We test the fiberoptic light probe. We make final microscope adjustments, then adjust the height and position of the surgeon's chair so that the surgeon is sitting with his or her back straight (to avoid later discomfort) and on the front edge of the chair (to avoid later pressure-induced numbness of the feet). Ideally, the angle between the surgeon's upper leg and lower leg approximates 90 degrees. All foot pedals should be functional and comfortably accessible. The infusion bottle height is adjusted to about 13–15 cm above the level of the eye.

The operating microscope should have coaxial illumination and X-Y function. A beam splitter is used to give the assistant a coaxial view. We use a microscope with a multifunctional foot switch that controls zoom, focus, X-Y movement, room lights, and operating microscope lights. We prefer to cover the microscope with a sterile plastic drape to avoid instrument contamination. We orient the microscope vertically to permit equal access to all meridians of the eye. Many microscopes can be tilted toward or away from the surgeon to improve visualization of the superior or inferior periphery. The microscope foot pedal should be draped with a plastic bag to prevent fluids from causing electrical malfunction.

Operative Technique

Entrance into the Eye

If a scleral buckle is planned, we open the conjunctiva 360 degrees at the limbus, and loop the muscles with 2-0 silk sutures. However, we do not create a full limbal peritomy if we do not plan on placing a scleral buckle. Figure 8-9 shows an eye prepared for vitrectomy when a scleral buckle is not planned. We place a transconjunctival 4-0 silk suture on DO-1 needle through the tendon of the medial rectus muscle. We then make a temporal conjunctival limbal peritomy with a radial relaxing incision at the temporal horizontal meridian. We expose the sclera and place a 4-0 silk traction suture through the tendon of the lateral rectus muscle, permitting good exposure for the temporal sclerotomy sites (Figure 8-9). We then make a 5-mm radial conjunctival incision that extends from the limbus nasally toward an area just superior to the medial rectus muscle. We apply light bipolar diathermy to the episcleral vessels in preparation for making the sclerotomies.

The ideal sclerotomy site is through the pars plana anterior to the vitreous base. Figure 8-10 shows the surgical anatomy between the limbus and the ora serrata. (The sclerotomy site is usually located between the anterior pars plana and the anterior vitreous base.) Sclerotomies are made 3 mm posterior to the limbus in aphakic or pseudophakic eyes or in eyes in which a lensectomy is planned. Sclerotomies are made 3.5–4.0 mm posterior to the limbus in phakic eyes. The sclerotomy sites must be made more anteriorly in infants' eyes and in eyes in which the retina is pulled anteriorly over the pars plana by anterior traction.

Sclerotomy sites should be close to the horizontal meridians in order to allow equal access of instruments to the superior and inferior peripheral retina, but we try to avoid the anterior ciliary arteries located anterior to the muscle insertions. The infusion port should be located just inferior to the meridian of the lateral rectus insertion, while the instrument sclerotomies should be just superior to the meridian of the horizontal rectus insertions, 150–160 degrees apart (Figure 8-9). Infusion ports or instruments placed too far from the horizontal meridian may hamper movement of the eye due to impaction of the instruments or the infusion tubing on the lid speculum. We mark

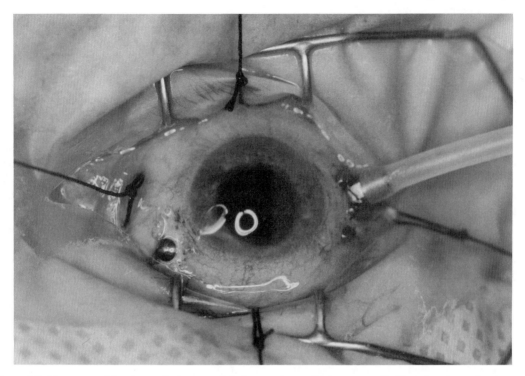

Figure 8-9. Eye prepared for vitreoretinal surgery. Infusion port inserted inferotemporally. Note plugs in nasal and temporal sclerotomies.

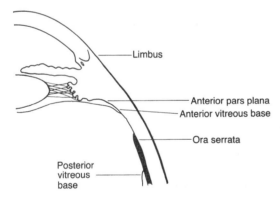

Figure 8-10. Surgical anatomy from limbus to posterior vitreous base.

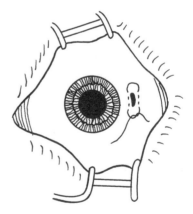

Figure 8-11. Mattress suture preplaced around sclerotomy prior to placement of infusion port.

the site of the planned sclerotomy with a marking pencil after measuring with calipers. We place a 5-0 nylon mattress suture on a DO-5 needle around the planned site of the infusion port (Figure 8-11). We make the sclerotomy with a 19-gauge microvitreoretinal blade (MVR blade) with the flat portion parallel to the limbus. Alternatively, a 20-gauge MVR blade may be used and the opening dilated with a 19-gauge sharp needle. We direct the knife toward the center of the phakic eye, although it can be directed slightly more anteriorly in the aphakic or pseudophakic eye. The widest portion of the arrowhead-like knife must pass through the pars plana epithelium. This is accomplished by passing the tip approximately 5 mm into the eye. We flush any remaining air bubbles from the infusion line; then, with the infusion turned off, the infusion cannula is inserted. We use a 4-mm long cannula in most eyes, but if the choroid is thickened, the pars plana is covered by dense blood, inflammatory cells, or fibrous tissue, or the pars plana is detached, a 6-mm cannula can be used in the aphakic or pseudophakic eye. The cannula is fixed in place with the mattress suture. If the tip of the infusion cannula does not pierce the pars plana epithelium, infusion into the choroidal or subretinal space may result. The tip is easily visualized by directing the fiberoptic light from the opposite side of the eye through the cornea as the infusion port is depressed into the eye. The tip should be clearly identified before the infusion is turned on. If blood, cataract, or other opacity obscures the tip of the cannula, a secondary hand-held, 20-gauge infusion needle, with the tip visually identified in the eye, should be used for infusion until the tip of the infusion cannula can be visualized.

We make the instrument sclerotomies with a 20-gauge rather than a 19-gauge MVR blade so that there is less leakage from the sites during vitrectomy. We usually make the nasal sclerotomy first for the fiberoptic light probe. We direct the light probe toward the center of the phakic eye, but it can be directed more anteriorly in the aphakic or pseudophakic eye. With the eye stabilized by the nasal instrument, we make the temporal sclerotomy, then place the vitrectomy instrument into the eye. In the aphakic eye, the instruments are easily visualized in the pupillary space without a contact lens. In the phakic eye, we place the contact lens on the eye immediately in order to identify the instruments. If one or both instruments cannot be seen, the surgeon should back his or her eyes away from the microscope and examine the eye grossly. Instruments can be realigned to point toward the center of the eye, then the tips can be more easily seen when the surgeon once again looks through the microscope. If tissue is seen to be pushed forward by either instrument, that instrument should be removed and the sclerotomy site opened once more with the MVR blade before the instrument is reinserted into the eye.

Basic Vitrectomy

The position of the wrist rest should be higher in the phakic eye to keep the hand position somewhat more anterior; thus, the instrument tips will be directed more posteriorly to avoid damage to the lens. In the phakic eye, the surgeon should develop a sense of hand position to avoid bringing the instruments anteriorly and possibly damaging the lens.

The eye is manipulated with a bimanual technique with the two instruments. The basic eye movements are vertical, horizontal, and oblique ductions of the eye. These movements are made by exerting equal force with the two instruments in the same direction. Unequal force or torsional forces by the instruments will create corneal striae and reduce visibility. Instruments are held with the fingertips. Individual instrument manipulations that must be mastered are rotational and in-out movements. Combinations of the bimanual manipulations of the eye and rotational and in-out movements are necessary to perform basic vitrectomy techniques.

The fiberoptic light should be held a short distance away from the vitrectomy instrument and directed just to the side or just beyond the tip of the instrument to illuminate the vitreous and reduce glare. Indirect illumination is frequently useful and is accomplished by directing light at the posterior retina and using the reflected light to illuminate the field.

Moderate suction (maximum of 150 mm Hg) and a rapid cutting rate (400–600 cycles per second or sometimes higher) are used. After ascertaining that the infusion is on, cutting is tested in the central anterior vitreous. With low suction, the vitreous is engaged in the port. If the instrument is not cutting adequately, the vitrectomy hand piece should be replaced. If there is inadequate suction or if suction does not disengage, the instrument console should be checked. Vitreous to be removed may be opaque or clear. If the vitreous is clear, the retina can be easily monitored during vitrectomy. If the vitreous is opaque, the retina is often hidden and there may be a risk of cutting into the retina.

The four basic vitreoretinal relationships are as follows: (1) vitreous separated from attached retina, (2) vitreous not separated from attached retina, (3) vitreous separated from detached retina, and (4) vitreous adherent to detached retina. In addition, there are eyes with partial vitreoretinal separation with focal or broad areas of vitreoretinal adhesion. The variable vitreoretinal relationships require different approaches during vitrectomy.

If the instrument is functioning properly, the vitrectomy is begun. Loose central vitreous not under traction will usually come directly toward the port. The instrument tip is placed in the anterior central vitreous and directed either slightly superiorly or inferiorly to begin the vitrectomy. The surgeon should follow the instrument tip with the X-Y of the operating microscope, always keeping the instruments in the center of the field. Frequent change of depth of focus anterior and posterior to the field of the instruments will keep the surgeon aware of any unwanted tissue, such as retina that might be coming toward the instrument. The instrument cuts best if the port is directed toward the vitreous to be cut (Figure 8-12A). If loose vitreous is not under traction, it will sometimes curl around the probe to the port when the port is directed away from the vitreous (and away from the retina). This is a good method if the retina cannot be seen. If the attached retina can be identified, direct cutting with the port directed toward the vitreous is preferable. If the vitreous is under traction, the port must be directed at the vitreous to be cut. In order to section a vitreous band, it must be directly engaged by the vitreous cutter. While cutting vitreous, the surgeon should disengage from the vitreous regularly to check that the instrument continues to cut well.

Clear vitreous may be difficult to visualize during cutting. Formed vitreous can be seen when directly illuminated with the fiberoptic light, but is difficult to see with diffuse or indirect illumination. If vitreous is not well seen, the angle or distance of the fiberoptic light from the vitreous should be adjusted in order to better illuminate the vitreous.

An important point in the procedure is the incision of the posterior hyaloid. This frequently provides the first view of the retina. The posterior hyaloid should first be opened over attached retina, if possible, and preferably in an area in which the vitreous is well separated from the retina. The preoperative ultrasound scan will frequently delineate the best area. If the posterior hyaloid is collapsed and thin, it may curl around the vitrectomy instrument tip into the cutting port even if the port is not directed toward the hyaloid. If the hyaloid is thickened, it is necessary to direct the port toward the hyaloid. The opening in the posterior hyaloid is enlarged until the retina can be visualized. If blood in the subhyaloid space obscures the retina, after the opening is adequately enlarged, the blood is removed with a silicone-tip suction needle. When the retina is well-visualized, the cutting port of the vitrectomy instrument is placed through the opening in the hyaloid and the port is directed away from the retina toward the hyaloidal edge. The hyaloid is engaged and cut, centrifugally enlarging the opening in progressively larger concentric circles toward the periphery. It is necessary to cut the peripheral vitreous back far enough to give an adequate view of the peripheral retina (Figure 8-12B). In eyes at risk of anterior cellular proliferation (eyes with retinal detachment, diabetes, or anterior retinal breaks) scleral depression is useful in exposing the peripheral vitreous for excision.

Removal of the peripheral vitreous is more difficult than removal of the posterior vitreous. The inexperienced surgeon may have difficulty visualizing

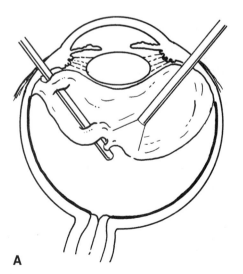
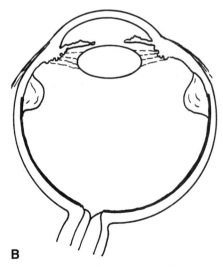

A   **B**

Figure 8-12. A, Cutting port directed toward vitreous to be cut. **B,** Postvitrectomy eye. Only remaining vitreous is at vitreous base.

the peripheral vitreous. There may be inadequate illumination and striae and distortion of the cornea created by unequal force on the instruments when taking the eye to extremes of direction. Relaxing the grip and equalizing the force on the instruments in order to reduce tension between the sclerotomy sites can eliminate the corneal striae.

Direct illumination of the peripheral vitreous on the side of the vitreous-cutting instrument is impossible in the phakic eye without touching the lens with the shaft of the fiberoptic light source (Figure 8-13A). Adequate illumination can be obtained by using indirect illumination, in which the light is directed toward the posterior retina using the reflected light for visualization (Figure 8-13B). The surgeon should not try to cut the far peripheral vitreous on the side opposite the entrance site of the cutting instrument because of the danger of touching the lens with the shaft of the instrument. That vitreous can best be removed by exchanging the instruments so that the cutting instrument is on the side of the peripheral vitreous to be cut. Remaining blood or debris on the retinal surface is removed with the silicone-tip suction needle.

If the retina is partially detached, the posterior hyaloid should be incised over attached retina if possible. If the retina is completely detached, the incision of the hyaloid is best done over a less bullous area. Although preoperative ultrasound scans may be helpful, the configuration of the retinal detachment may change at surgery, so an incision posteriorly over the optic nerve where the retina is flat is usually best. If the posterior hyaloid is collapsed anteriorly, the cutting port is directed anteriorly and the vitreous and posterior hyaloid may curl around the tip into the cutting port during suction. However, it is usually necessary to direct the cutting port at least parallel with the collapsed hyaloid or directly toward a thickened or taut hyaloid to create an opening. Cutting and suction should stop as soon as an opening is made in the hyaloid. Once the hyaloid is opened, the instrument tip is placed through the opening and the cutting port is directed away from the detached retina toward the hyaloid. Low suction is applied and the retina is kept in view during vitrectomy. Vitreous is cut peripherally toward the vitreous base. In the periphery there is danger of suctioning bullous retina into the cutting tip. A good method to use in the periphery near the retina is to engage the vitreous with low suction and short bursts of cutting, letting the vitreous (and retina) fall back between cuts. If a retinal break is located, subretinal fluid can be aspirated with the silicone-tip suction needle to partially flatten the retina, thus reducing the risk of peripheral retinal damage. Newer high-speed vitreous cutting instruments may exert less traction on the detached retina because there is less unobstructed suction between

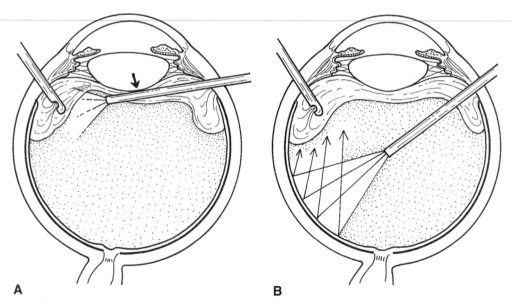

A   **B**

Figure 8-13. A, Lens touch with endoilluminator while illuminating vitreous on opposite side of eye. **B,** Indirect illumination of vitreous avoids lens touch.

the high-speed cuts. There is more control during the procedure because of the reduced mobility of the retina during cutting.

Another maneuver that will reduce the mobility of the detached retina is to inject perfluorocarbon liquid (PFCL) over the posterior pole to flatten the retina posterior to the peripheral vitreous. It is important that posterior vitreous and membranes be removed prior to PFCL injection and that there be no remaining posterior retinal traction. The PFCL should not extend over retinal breaks still under traction because of the risk of the PFCL going beneath the retina. The PFCL should not extend so far anteriorly so as to flatten the peripheral vitreous against the retina. Vitreous should be cut as far peripherally as safety permits. In most cases of retinal detachment, scleral depression (usually by an assistant with a scleral depressor or with a cotton-tipped applicator) should be performed during cutting to improve visibility and access to the peripheral vitreous. During scleral depression there is risk of inadvertent retinal damage by the instruments. During initial placement of the external scleral depressor, the internal instruments should be kept well clear of the area of depression. Once the depressor is in place, the assistant should not change the position of the scleral depressor until the surgeon requests a change and moves the internal instruments out of the way. At the central area of depression the retina is pushed inwardly toward the vitreous, so it is often safest to cut at the margin of the area of depression. A contact or noncontact wide-angle viewing system reduces the need for scleral depression during excision of the peripheral vitreous.

In some cases of rhegmatogenous retinal detachment, diabetic retinopathy, penetrating ocular injury, retained intraocular foreign body, uveitis, or epiretinal membrane, the posterior cortical vitreous may not be separated from the retina. In most cases it is best to surgically separate the vitreous, which, if left in contact with the retina, may act as a scaffold for proliferation of scar tissue. In addition, it is necessary to separate the posterior cortical vitreous from the retina in cases of macular hole. Sometimes as the formed central vitreous is cut, the posterior hyaloid will spontaneously separate from the retina. In most cases, however, it is necessary to separate the posterior hyaloid mechanically. If the vitreous is clear, it is sometimes difficult to determine if the hyaloid is separated. As the posterior cortical vitreous is cut, one can often see traction causing movement of the retina beneath the vitreous being cut. If the vitreous is densely opaque, visualization of the vitreoretinal junction may be difficult. By "shaving" the vitreous in layers with low suction and approaching the retina over the optic nerve area, the junction can usually be visualized safely. By approaching over the optic nerve, there is less risk of engaging a detached retina.

The vitreous can be separated from the retina by one of two methods. We first apply suction to the cortical vitreous over the optic nerve head border (Figure 8-14). It is best to begin the maneuver before the core (central) vitrectomy is complete, because at that stage the vitreous is easier to engage. By gradually increasing suction with a silicone-tip needle anterior to the edge of the optic nerve head, the posterior cortical vitreous can usually be elevated. The vitrectomy instrument can be used in a similar manner (with suction only) facing the open port posteriorly. Higher levels of suction are frequently required (up to 200 mm Hg). Once the vitreous is elevated from the optic disc, fluid will go into the subhyaloid space through the opening over the optic nerve head to create, in effect, a rhegmatogenous separation of the vitreous. A membrane pick can then be used to help separate the vitreous out to the retinal periphery (Figure 8-15). In the rare event that the posterior cortical vitreous will not

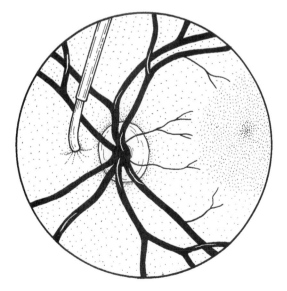

Figure 8-14. "Fish-strike sign" as aspiration through silicone-tip needle engages posterior vitreous cortex and causes torsion of needle tip.

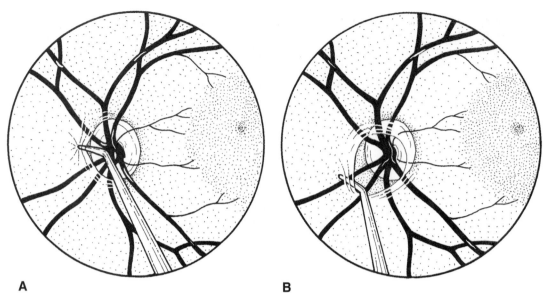

Figure 8-15. A, B, Lifting and separating posterior hyaloid with pick placed through epipapillary opening.

separate with suction, a sharp membrane pick can be used to separate the hyaloid (Figure 8-16). A sharp but short-tipped pick is best and we have found the MVR blade useful. We create a short barb of the tip by pushing it against a flat metal surface while observing the tip with the operating microscope. By

scratching the surface of the hyaloid at the optic nerve head edge, we engage the hyaloid and lift it away from the retina. The hyaloid then separates in a manner similar to that described with the suction technique. If the retina is detached, it is best to fixate the retina gently with a second instrument (i.e., the light

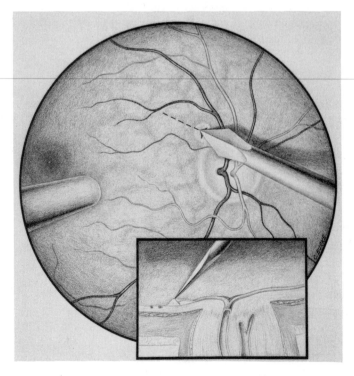

Figure 8-16. Separation of posterior hyaloid with sharp pick. Vitreous engaged at edge of optic disc.

probe or an illuminated spatula) as the hyaloid is separated. As the hyaloid is stripped to the periphery, the surgeon should constantly assess whether there is excess vitreoretinal traction (which might lead to retinal tearing or hemorrhage). If the vitreous will not separate from a firm vitreoretinal adhesion, the vitreous should be separated and circumcised around the adhesion. Figure 8-17 shows the vitreous being cut with the vitreous cutter around a point of adhesion to relieve the traction.

Termination of the Procedure

When the instruments are removed from the eye, the infusion should be turned off to prevent incarceration of vitreous and retina in the wound. Scleral plugs should be placed in the sclerotomy sites, and the intraocular pressure restored to normal with the infusion.

The eye should be examined with the indirect ophthalmoscope to determine whether adequate vitreous was removed and to look for complications. The peripheral retina should be examined with scleral depression to search for dialyses or tears at the vitreous base and posterior to the instrument sites.

With the infusion off, one plug is removed, and incarcerated vitreous is removed with the vitreous cutting instrument, using low suction. Remaining vitreous is engaged with a dry cellulose sponge and cut with scissors at the lips of the wound. When all gross

vitreous has been removed from the wound, the sclerotomy is closed with a figure-of-eight 7-0 suture. The remaining sclerotomy sites are closed in a similar manner. The pressure is adjusted if necessary with BSS injected through the limbus in the aphakic eye or through the pars plana in the phakic eye. The conjunctiva is closed with 6-0 plain gut or 7-0 Vicryl sutures.

Lensectomy

Lensectomy is performed if lens opacification will prevent adequate visualization during vitrectomy. Rarely, the lens may opacify during surgery and require a lensectomy. A clear lens may be removed during surgery for certain complicated retinal detachments (such as cases requiring membrane dissection in the vicinity of the vitreous base). The lens is removed most easily at the beginning of the procedure, so the decision for lensectomy should be made preoperatively if possible. Posterior subcapsular opacities interfere the most with visualization. Adequate visualization is possible through moderate nuclear sclerosis and cortical opacities.

The hardness of the nucleus is graded preoperatively. Nuclear sclerosis is graded on a 0–4+ scale. A 4+ nuclear sclerotic lens is very hard, frequently brunescent, and the lens is prominently seen in retroillumination. We remove lenses with up to 3+ nuclear sclerosis with pars plana ultrasound

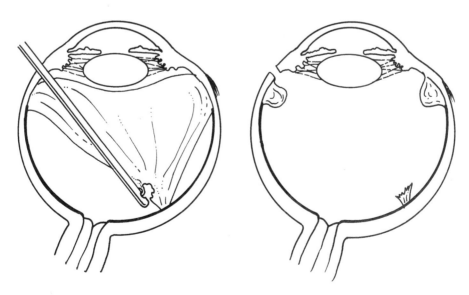

Figure 8-17. Circumcision of vitreous around focal vitreoretinal adhesion.

fragmentation, and those with 4+ nuclear sclerosis are removed by limbal extraction.

If limbal extraction is necessary, we perform an extracapsular extraction of the nucleus. We close the limbal wound with interrupted 10-0 nylon sutures and then remove the remainder of the lens cortex and capsule during the pars plana vitrectomy.

For pars plana ultrasound fragmentation, after the infusion port has been sutured in place, the temporal sclerotomy is made as usual, directed toward the center of the vitreous cavity. Then the MVR blade is redirected through the equator of the lens into the nucleus. The sharp MVR blade will easily cut into a moderately hard nucleus, but may partially dislocate a very hard nucleus. Nuclear movement should be carefully observed to judge hardness. The ultrasound needle is placed into the lens through the sclerotomy site.

After the nasal sclerotomy is made, we place a 20-gauge infusion needle through the nasal equator of the lens. We bend the needle approximately 30 degrees, 5–7 mm from the tip because the bend permits better access across the patient's nose. We temporarily interrupt the pars plana infusion by clamping the infusion tubing and attach the infusion to the 20-gauge needle. We turn on the infusion in the center of the lens and begin ultrasound fragmentation of the nucleus with the infusion needle near but not touching the ultrasound needle (Figure 8-18A).

It is important to initiate a flow of fluid through the ultrasound needle at the beginning of the lensectomy so that nuclear material does not obstruct the tip. Ultrasound is applied in short bursts so as not to generate heat with prolonged activation. The nucleus is removed inside out, preserving the cortex until the end, to help fixate the nucleus. Anterior, posterior, and peripheral nucleus are progressively removed with intermittent simultaneous ultrasound fragmentation and suction. After the nucleus is removed, the cortex can be aspirated with the ultrasound needle without ultrasound energy (Figure 8-18B). The peripheral cortex is stripped from behind the iris by engaging and gently pulling cortex toward the center of the pupil with simultaneous suction. If the ante-

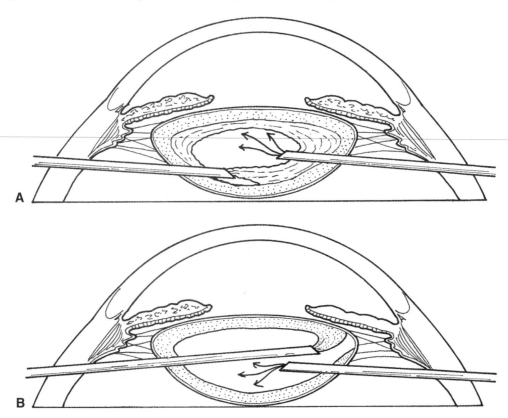

Figure 8-18. Pars plana lensectomy. **A,** Ultrasound fragmentation of nucleus of lens from inside-out. **B,** Aspiration and stripping of residual lens cortex.

rior capsule remains intact, there is little danger of engaging iris. Nevertheless, the instrument tip should not be pointed directly at the iris.

We usually remove the whole lens capsule in the following manner. We remove the central portion of the anterior capsule, leaving a rim of capsule seen through the pupil. We then place a vitreoretinal forcep in one of the sclerotomies and grasp the edge of the remaining anterior capsule and pull it centrally to expose the peripheral lens capsule and the zonules. We then cut the zonules with the automated scissors (MPC, Alcon, Fort Worth). It is possible to section all of the zonules with the scissors and remove the remaining capsule, although it is usually necessary to change sclerotomy sites with the instruments to access all of the zonules.

Alternatively, the anterior capsule can be left in place to support a posterior chamber intraocular lens. A central 5 mm opening is usually made in the anterior capsule to improve subsequent visualization during the remainder of the vitrectomy procedure. If during lensectomy the posterior capsule is prematurely broken, there is risk of posterior dislocation of lens material. Lens nucleus or cortex will usually rest on the intact vitreous and can be engaged and fragmented. The infusion needle can be used to support loose fragments, but the two needles should not touch because metallic fragments may be released. If a lens fragment falls posteriorly, we remove anterior lens material as described above with the ultrasound needle, the vitrectomy instrument, or both. We then perform a vitrectomy with the vitrectomy instrument. Following vitrectomy, we once more place the ultrasound needle in the eye, and remove the posterior lens material with posterior ultrasound fragmentation. Figure 8-19A shows the posterior lens fragment engaged with suction from the ultrasound fragmentation needle. The ultrasound is activated after the fragment is taken to the midvitreous cavity. Soft nuclei mold to enter the tip of the needle, but harder nuclei fracture into smaller pieces. Each fragment is then removed individually. It is important that ultrasound not be activated near the retinal surface because of the risk of retinal damage.

Additional Techniques in Vitreous Surgery

Membrane Peeling

Indications

Membrane peeling is done to remove epiretinal membranes. Epiretinal membranes may be idiopathic or may be associated with a variety of disorders, including proliferative vitreoretinopathy,

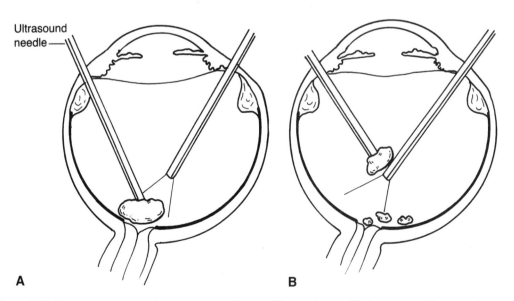

Ultrasound needle

A   **B**

Figure 8-19. Ultrasound fragmentation of posteriorly dislocated lens nucleus. **A,** Nucleus retrieved from retinal surface with suction without ultrasound. **B,** Nucleus fragmented with ultrasound in midvitreous cavity. Adapted from Lewis JM, Abrams GW, Werner JC. Management of complicated retinal detachment. In: Albert DM, ed. *Ophthalmic Surgery: Principles and Practice.* Vol. 1. Malden, MA: Blackwell Science; 1999:1306.

proliferative vascular retinopathy, uveitis, and trauma.

Instrumentation

Instruments used for membrane removal are picks and forceps. Several varieties of sharp or blunt picks or spatulas are manufactured. Forceps are usually of the end-opening variety and several are available (see Figure 8-5).

Surgical Technique

Epiretinal Membrane with Attached Retina. Most epiretinal membranes removed in the presence of an attached retina involve the macula. The retina beneath the membrane is usually folded. There is sometimes a thickened, elevated, or rolled edge to the membrane but the edge may be flat and difficult to see. In most cases the edge of the membrane is engaged with a pick and elevated (Figure 8-20A). We use a sharp, barb-like pick that we create under the microscope by bending the tip of the 20-gauge MVR blade against the flat handle of another instrument. There are also commercially available sharp membrane picks. We engage the edge of the membrane and elevate it with a stripping motion. Sometimes the membrane will strip free with the pick, but usually it must be grasped with vitreoretinal forceps (Figure 8-20B). A fine, end-grabbing forceps is best for this task because the membrane and retina are not obscured by the forceps and can be easily visualized as the membrane is grasped.

The retina beneath the membrane is often whitened by axoplasmic stasis in the nerve fiber layer. This may resemble additional membranes, but usually no further membrane is present. Unless further membrane clearly remains, attempts at further membrane stripping should be avoided. The retinal thickening and whitening will resolve postoperatively.

Epiretinal Membranes with Retinal Detachment. Epiretinal membranes associated with proliferative vitreoretinopathy may be widespread. Membranes are often associated with fixed folds, star folds, and marked wrinkling and contraction. Membranes may not be readily seen but should be expected in the center of a star fold or at the anterior extent of a fixed radial fold. The only sign of some membranes is a graying of the retinal surface. Abrupt disappearance of a retinal vessel often indicates a fold obscured by an epiretinal membrane. Immature membranes may be composed of a sheet of contractile proliferative cells, with little collagenous matrix, while mature membranes contain an abundant collagenous matrix. Mature membranes do not tear as easily as immature membranes and are more easily stripped free.

We usually begin membrane stripping posteriorly at the optic nerve head and progress anteriorly. The posterior retina is thicker than the anterior retina and is fixed at the optic nerve; therefore, membrane peeling posteriorly to anteriorly is both safer and easier.

Using a 30-degree fiberoptic illuminated pick, we elevate the edge of the membrane (Figure 8-21A).

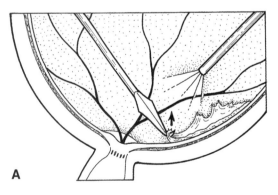
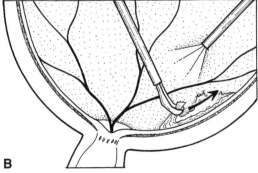

Figure 8-20. Epiretinal membrane removal—attached retina. **A,** Membrane edge lifted with membrane pick. **B,** Membrane grasped and removed with vitreous forcep. Traction force parallel with retinal surface. Adapted from Lewis JM, Abrams GW, Werner JC. Management of complicated retinal detachment. In: Albert DM, ed. *Ophthalmic Surgery: Principles and Practice.* Vol. 1. Malden, MA: Blackwell Science; 1999:1307.

We then grasp the membrane with forceps. We recommend a bimanual technique be used for membrane removal. With the membrane under tension by the forceps, we use the illuminated pick to hold the retina back during stripping (Figure 8-21B) or, alternatively, as a spatula to help free the membrane from the retina. It is useful to run the illuminated pick or barbed MVR blade within retinal folds (Figure 8-22A) in order to locate membranes. At a star fold, we often engage the membrane in the center by running the illuminated pick radially in a fold toward the center of the star fold (Figure 8-22B). It is important to monitor the surrounding retina when stripping a membrane because large breaks can occur in a retina under traction. The risk of retinal tearing is reduced by using a bimanual technique, in which the retina is held back with another instrument such as the fiberoptic illuminated pick or spatula during membrane peeling. Thin or tight membranes are sometimes difficult to engage with a blunt pick. These can often be engaged with the short, sharp pick produced by barbing the tip of the MVR blade. We do not use the barbed MVR blade for routine membrane peeling because the sharp blade increases the risk of internal limiting membrane damage or tearing of the retina.

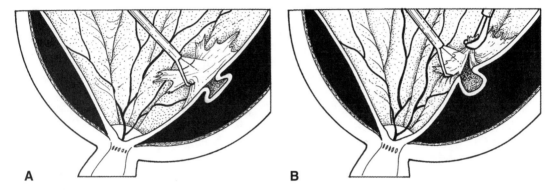

Figure 8-21. Epiretinal membrane removal—detached retina. **A,** Large membrane bridges retinal fold. Membrane edge lifted with illuminated pick. **B,** Membrane grasped and removed with vitreous forcep. Retinal countertraction with illuminated pick during membrane removal.

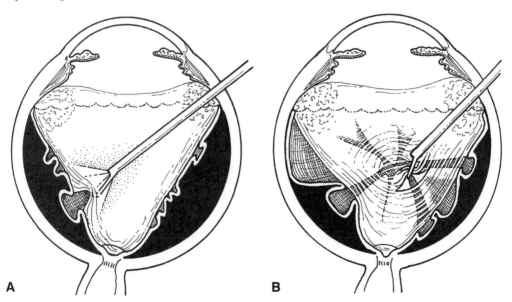

Figure 8-22. Membrane removal—PVR. **A,** Membrane engaged in retinal fold with illuminated pick. **B,** Membrane engaged with pick in center of "star fold."

Peripheral Membrane Removal. Peripheral vitreoretinal membranes are found most commonly in proliferative vitreoretinopathy or following ocular trauma, but are sometimes found associated with proliferative vascular retinopathies. Most peripheral membranes are associated with the vitreous base area. The most severe forms of anterior proliferative vitreoretinopathy are found following previous vitreous surgery. There are two major forms of anterior PVR: circumferential contraction caused by contraction of membranes formed on the peripheral retina, usually at the posterior edge of the vitreous base; and anterior retinal displacement, once called "anterior loop contraction." This latter form of PVR is caused by fibrous proliferation on the surface of the vitreous base with contraction that leads to traction retinal detachment and anterior displacement of the peripheral retina. Figure 8-23A shows an eye with proliferative vitreoretinopathy with proliferation of cells on remaining peripheral vitreous following vitrectomy. Following contraction of the vitreous base, the anterior retina is pulled forward toward the pars plana (Figure 8-23B), the ciliary body, or even the posterior iris surface. Anterior fibrovascular proliferation can be found following diabetic vitrectomy with either fibrous proliferation and contraction from a sclerotomy site or severe fibrovascular proliferation from the peripheral retina called "anterior hyaloidal fibrovascular proliferation." While anterior proliferative membranes in diabetic retinopathy tend to be more vascular, the appearance of the peripheral retina is similar to that found in anterior retinal displacement.

Surgical Technique

Surgical dissection in the vitreous base area necessitates removal of the lens. It is recommended that the lens capsule, which may become involved in anterior fibrous proliferation, be completely removed (as mentioned above). Scleral depression is used to allow visualization of the vitreous base. Wide iris dilatation is helpful. Iris retractors may be useful if the pupil is miotic. Coaxial illumination is used for the anterior portion of the dissection. While depressing the anterior vitreous into view, the vitrectomy instrument is used to remove any remaining formed vitreous (Figure 8-24).

Circumferential contraction becomes apparent as membranes are peeled from posteriorly to anteriorly. There are usually diffuse membranes and vitreous is often adherent to these membranes, especially throughout the inferior 180 degrees of the retina. The vitreous and the membranes should be stripped anteriorly to the vitreous base. Once the membranes have been stripped anteriorly and removed if possible, the vitreous is excised to the retinal surface at the vitreous base with the vitreous cutter utilizing scleral depression.

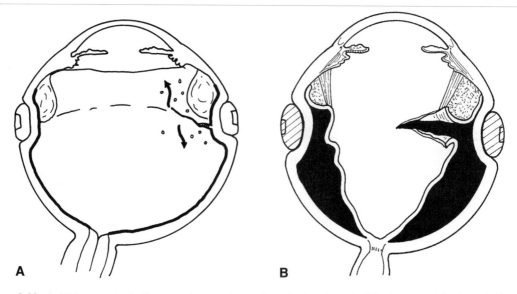

A   **B**

Figure 8-23. A, Disbursement of cells onto retina and vitreous base. **B,** Anterior retinal displacement. Membrane bridging vitreous base pulls anterior retina toward pars plana.

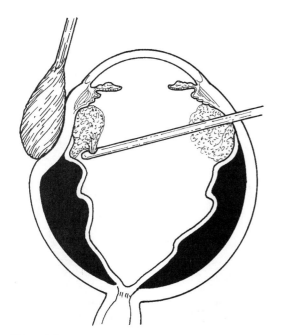

Figure 8-24. Removal of vitreous at vitreous base while depressing the sclera.

of the vitreous base may be uncovered in the trough after the membrane is opened and should be cut to the surface of the peripheral retina and pars plana using the vitreous cutting instrument.

The circumferential component of anterior retinal displacement is released by either excising the membrane on the surface of the vitreous base using bimanual dissection or making multiple radial cuts in the membrane. When using coaxial illumination, it is possible to use both forceps and scissors in a bimanual dissection technique. For endoillumination during bimanual dissection, the fiberoptic illuminated pick or spatula is useful. Fiberoptic illuminated forceps and scissors have been introduced, but have not been universally adopted because of their expense and limited availability. These illuminated instruments are helpful during bimanual dissection of the vitreous base.

Anterior retinal displacement may only be apparent by a gray membrane that covers the tightly contracted vitreous base. The anterior retina is often pulled forward but may be obscured. There are two components to the anterior retinal displacement and each must be dealt with. Circumferential sectioning of a membrane that covers the vitreous base is necessary to relieve an anterior-posterior (AP) component that pulls the retina anteriorly. A circumferential component of contraction that pulls the retina centrally and causes radial folds that extend posteriorly, must also be relieved.

The tight capsule-like membrane that overlies the vitreous base is incised with the tip of a sharp blade such as the MVR blade. After an opening is created in this membrane, vertically cutting scissors, such as the membrane peeler-cutter (MPC) scissors (Alcon Laboratories, Fort Worth), are used to section the membrane anterior to the anterior extent of the retina in a circumferential direction (Figure 8-25). A bimanual technique is often useful and a fiberoptic illuminated pick or spatula can be used to retract the fibrous membrane away from the vitreous base as it is cut. The anterior retinal displacement is usually most prominent in the inferior 180 degrees but can extend 360 degrees. There may be a "trough" created by the membrane between the anterior and posterior edges of the membrane (see Figure 8-25). Formed vitreous

Treatment of Retinal Breaks and Retinal Detachment

Retinal breaks may be present prior to vitreous surgery or may occur as a result of membrane

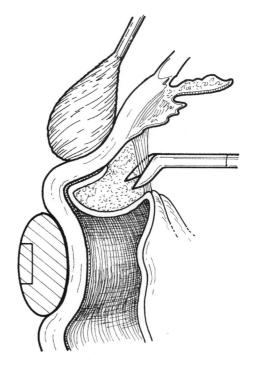

Figure 8-25. Treatment of anterior retinal displacement by section of membrane overlying vitreous base.

removal techniques. Retinal detachment in association with the retinal breaks is usually treated with a combination of internal (vitrectomy) and external (scleral buckling) techniques. It is necessary to relieve all traction from the retinal breaks. It is best to remove remaining membranes by membrane peeling or excision, but sectioning of the membranes is sometimes adequate. The retinal breaks are marked with endodiathermy. The endodiathermy will whiten the edges of the break and will allow easy identification following fluid-air exchange. Subretinal fluid may be drained internally during fluid-air exchange through a posterior retinal break if present. A continuous infusion air pump is used during fluid-air exchange. The air pump is attached to the infusion port. A silicone-tip suction needle is used to remove the intraocular fluid. For visualization, a –98.00-diopter biconcave contact lens is used in the phakic eye and the planoconcave contact lens is used in the aphakic eye. Alternatively, a wide-angle viewing system can be used during the exchange providing a superior view. During the initial portion of the fluid-air exchange, the eye is positioned so that the posterior drainage break is easily seen. It is often best to aspirate some anterior fluid and fill the anterior vitreous cavity with air. This gives a minified view of the fundus and it is necessary to refocus the microscope and increase the magnification. The drainage needle tip is then placed just anterior to or through the retinal break, and suction is applied (Figure 8-26). As the eye fills with air, a meniscus can be seen between the fluid posteriorly and the air anteriorly. When the fluid meniscus is posterior near the area of the retinal break, it is often best to use a "dripping" technique to remove the fluid. The drainage needle tip is placed over the drainage retinotomy and a bright reflex appears as the tip enters the fluid meniscus. The suction is applied until the fluid level drops below the needle tip and the reflex disappears. By continuing to "dip" over and into the break, the retina is completely flattened and as the needle tip enters the break, all of the subretinal fluid is removed without danger of the needle tip contacting the pigment epithelium and choroid. It is necessary to continue dipping over the retinotomy and the optic nerve for several minutes because fluid tends to continue to accumulate posteriorly for a short period of time. If a posterior break is not present, subretinal fluid can be drained through a more anterior retinal break using the cannulated extrusion instrument. PFCL over the posterior pole can be useful during this maneuver.

After the retina is completely flattened and all fluid has been removed, laser endophotocoagulation is applied to surround any retinal breaks (Figure 8-27).

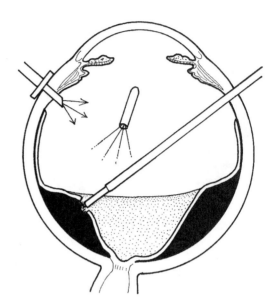

Figure 8-26. Fluid-air exchange. Aspiration of subretinal fluid through posterior break while air is simultaneously insufflated into the eye.

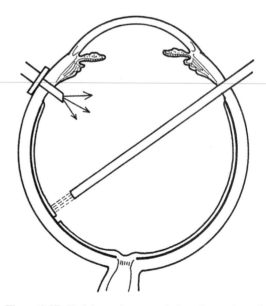

Figure 8-27. Endolaser photocoagulation of posterior retinal break in air-filled eye. Adapted from Lewis JM, Abrams GW, Werner JC. Management of complicated retinal detachment. In: Albert DM, ed. *Ophthalmic Surgery: Principles and Techniques.* Vol. 1. Malden, MA, Blackwell Science; 1999:542.

Perfluorocarbon Liquids

If a posterior break is not available and it is necessary to reattach the retina completely, we now rarely create a posterior retinotomy. In most instances, if a posterior break is not present for drainage of subretinal fluid, perfluorocarbon liquid (PFCL) is used to reattach the retina. PFCL is a synthetic liquid that is heavier than water or saline and will displace subretinal fluid anteriorly and reattach the retina from posteriorly to anteriorly. Perfluorocarbon liquid can be injected over the posterior pole after posterior membranes have been removed to flatten and stabilize the posterior retina. The heavy liquid flattening of the posterior retina makes midperipheral and far peripheral membrane peeling easier by reducing the mobility of the retina during membrane peeling (Figure 8-28A). As the retina is reattached with PFCL, fluid will egress through anterior retinal breaks into the vitreous cavity and allow near complete reattachment of the retina if the vitreous cavity is filled with PFCL (Figure 8-28B). The PFCL should never be directed toward a retinal break during injection because the PFCL stream will go into the subretinal space through the break. If PFCL is to be used, it is important that all traction be released before the level of PFCL is extended over a retinal break, otherwise the PFCL, which has a low interfacial surface tension, will go through the break into the subretinal space. However, once traction is relieved from the retina, it is safe to extend the PFCL level anterior to a retinal break (Figure 8-28C). Once the retina is attached, the PFCL can

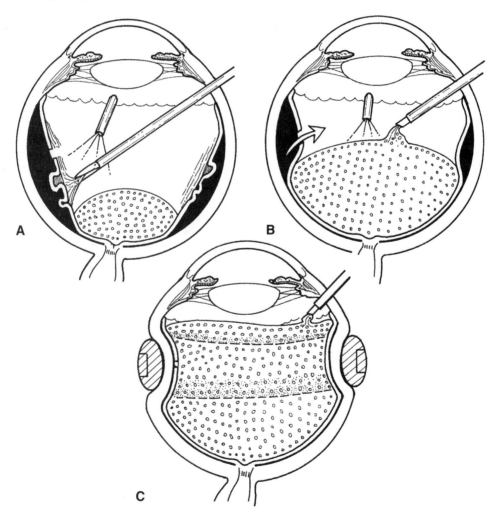

Figure 8-28. Perfluorocarbon liquid (PFCL) in treatment of PVR. **A,** PFCL holds posterior retina in place as midperipheral membrane is stripped. **B,** Retina reattached with PFCL. Subretinal fluid forced through retinal break into vitreous cavity. **C,** Retina completely reattached with PFCL. Scleral buckle in place.

be removed by a PFCL-air exchange. The PFCL is aspirated with a silicone-tip suction needle as the eye is simultaneously filled with air. If anterior subretinal fluid remains before PFCL-air exchange, it is desirable to aspirate subretinal fluid during the early portion of the exchange through an anterior retinal break so no subretinal fluid is forced posteriorly into the posterior pole by the air. While perfluoro-*n*-octane, the most commonly used PFCL has a high vapor pressure and will evaporate in air at body temperature, other commonly used PFCLs do not evaporate. Therefore, it is necessary to place a small amount of BSS over the posterior pole following PFCL-air exchange to cause coalescence of any remaining PFCL into bubbles that can be seen and aspirated. Because larger amounts of perfluoro-*n*-octane may not evaporate, we recommend flushing the posterior retina with BSS following use of any PFCL. Perfluorocarbon liquids are also useful for management of giant retinal tears and retinotomies (see following sections "Relaxing Retinotomies and Retinectomies" and "Giant Retinal Tears").

Scleral Buckling

A scleral buckle is only necessary in the presence of persistent or potential peripheral traction following vitrectomy. A detailed discussion of scleral buckling surgery is presented in Chapter 7. A scleral buckle is placed in most cases of proliferative vitreoretinopathy where there is often at least mild peripheral traction remaining and in many other cases of rhegmatogenous retinal detachment or giant retinal breaks. The sutures for the scleral buckle are most easily placed at the beginning of the case before starting the vitrectomy procedure. We prefer an encircling 4.0-mm diameter band (42 band) for most retinal detachments at vitrectomy that require a scleral buckle. Occasionally, if the vitreous base extends extremely posteriorly, we use a broader element such as a 7-mm diameter tire. If traction can be adequately relieved with vitrectomy, radial scleral buckling elements are usually not placed to support posterior retinal breaks. If it is not possible to relieve traction adequately, posterior radial buckles associated with an encircling element can be used to relieve posterior traction.

Relaxing Retinotomies and Retinectomies

Indications

Relaxing retinotomies and retinectomies (in which the retina is cut or excised) are used in the presence of shortening of the retina due to retinal incarceration or fibrous proliferation and contraction that prevents contact of the retina with the retinal pigment epithelium. Less significant, usually peripheral, retina is cut or removed to preserve function of posterior, more visually significant retina. A retinotomy is the act of cutting the retina to relax a shortened retina. A retinectomy is the actual excision of retina and associated proliferative membranes. Relaxing retinotomies and retinectomies should be performed only if other methods have failed or have no chance of success. Several ground rules are necessary in surgery utilizing relaxing retinotomies or retinectomies. The retinotomy or retinectomy should be performed late in the procedure, following complete membrane removal. If the retina is cut or excised prior to complete membrane removal, further membrane removal will be more difficult and may result in larger than necessary retinal defects or residual membranes that will lead to redetachment of the retina. As a general rule, a relaxing retinotomy (in which the retina is cut, but not excised) is made if the retina remains shortened after complete membrane removal; retinectomy (to excise membranes and involved retina) is performed if membranes remain and traction cannot be relieved by a scleral buckle. Larger peripheral retinotomies are less functionally significant than smaller posterior retinotomies. Although a larger peripheral retinotomy may be more difficult to manage, the greater preservation of retinal function is usually worthwhile. Circumferential relaxing retinotomies are usually preferred over radial retinotomies. In the face of circumferential traction, a radial retinotomy that adequately relieves traction may extend too far posteriorly into central retina.

Surgical Method

In most cases, the area of retinotomy is made posterior to the area of shortened, contracted retina (Figure 8-29A). Heavy diathermy is applied to the retinal vessels and light diathermy is applied along the area to be cut. The incision in retina is usually made with scissors (Figure 8-29A). To insure that no traction remains at the margins of the retinotomy, the retinotomy should be extended beyond the area of contraction into noncontracted retina on each end of the retinotomy. Figure 8-29B shows extension of the retinotomy anteriorly obliquely at each end of the retinotomy with excision (retinectomy) of the anterior contracted retina.

Retinectomy is usually done when membranes cannot be adequately removed from extremely contracted retina. Figure 8-30A shows contracted retina between two large retinal breaks. A retinectomy

should only be done if the retina cannot be reattached by other methods. To perform a retinectomy, diathermy is applied to the area of contracted retina and extended just into normal retina surrounding the area of contraction. Excision is usually done with the vitrectomy cutting instrument. Figure 8-30B shows a large retinal defect but traction is relieved and the retina is reattached.

There are several potentially serious complications of retinotomies and retinectomies. The major complications are hemorrhage, inability to unfold and reattach the retina, hypotony, visual field loss,

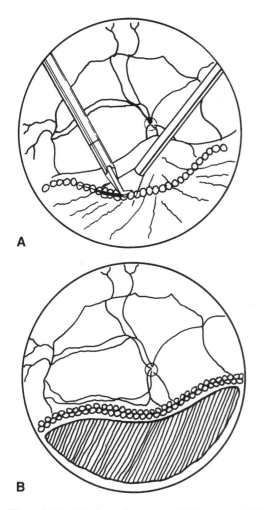

A

B

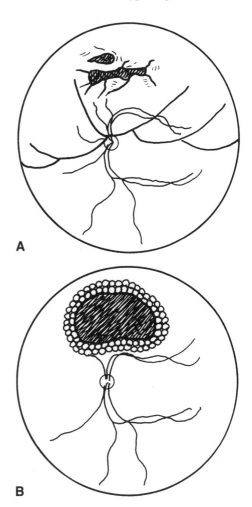

A

B

Figure 8-29. Relaxing retinotomy. **A,** Diathermy applied to peripheral retina on posterior edge of contracted retina. Blood vessels occluded with diathermy prior to retinotomy. **B,** Retinotomy followed by excision of scarred retina anterior to retinotomy. Retinotomy extended into normal retina beyond area of contracted retina.

Figure 8-30. A, Superior retinal breaks within area of contracted retina. **B,** Retinectomy of focally contracted retina. Laser treatment of edges of retinotomy. Adapted from Lewis JM, Abrams GW, Werner JC. Management of complicated retinal detachment. In: Albert DM, ed. *Ophthalmic Surgery: Principles and Techniques.* Vol. 1. Malden, MA, Blackwell Science; 1999:547.

recurrent fibrous proliferation from the retinotomy site, and persistent traction leading to retinal detachment when the retinotomy is too small. While careful planning and technique will prevent some of the complications, the potential seriousness of the complications means that relaxing retinotomy and retinectomy techniques should be used only if other techniques are unsuccessful.

Once the retinotomy is made, the retina may fold posteriorly like a giant retinal tear. It is best to make the retinotomy with the posterior retina held in place by PFCL, with the retinal incision anterior to the level of the PFCL. Once all traction is relieved and hemostasis is achieved, more PFCL is injected until the level of the PFCL is anterior to the margin of the retinotomy. We usually do laser treatment with PFCL in the eye, then remove the PFCL with a PFCL-air exchange. There is a risk of slippage of the edge of the retinotomy posteriorly during the PFCL-air exchange. In order to prevent slippage, it is important to "dry" the edge of the retinotomy before proceeding with the PFCL-air exchange. We dry the edge by holding the soft silicone tip of the backflush brush just anterior to the edge of the retinotomy in the initial portion of the PFCL-air exchange. This allows removal of fluid that may collect beneath the edge. If not removed, this fluid can be pushed posteriorly by the air and force the edge of the retina posteriorly, creating folds posterior to the edge of the retinotomy. Alternatively, a PFCL-silicone oil exchange can be done instead of a PFCL-air exchange. There is less risk of slippage of the flap with the PFCL-silicone oil exchange.

Intraocular Gases

Intraocular gases are used in vitreous surgery to tamponade retinal breaks. In eyes without significant retinal traction, air, which only persists in the eye for a few days, is useful. In eyes with tractional complications, gases that persist in the eye longer than air are useful for a prolonged retinal tamponade. The longer-acting gases are useful for two purposes: (1) to tamponade retinal breaks until an adhesion forms between the retina and the retinal pigment epithelium, and (2) to provide "retinal tamponade," in which the retina is held in place against the retinal pigment epithelium until widespread laser photocoagulation adhesions form. The latter indication has found widespread application with the use of long-acting gases in the treatment of proliferative vitreoretinopathy. In eyes with proliferative vitreoretinopathy, there is often minor retinal traction remaining following removal of epiretinal membranes. Sometimes a long-acting gas bubble can overcome minor residual epiretinal traction until the retina becomes permanently adherent to the underlying tissue following photocoagulation.

Besides air, the major gases used are sulfur hexafluoride (SF_6) and perfluoropropane (PFP or C_3F_8). An effective gas bubble is one that fills at least 50% of the vitreous cavity, which will maintain tamponade of the inferior retina when the patient is in the prone position. An eye filled with air will maintain an effective gas fill for only a few days. An eye filled with SF_6 will maintain an effective tamponade for approximately 7–10 days. An eye filled with C_3F_8 gas will maintain an effective tamponade for at least 3 weeks or more.

Longer-acting gases have in common a high molecular weight, low diffusion coefficient, and low water solubility. When these gases are injected in a pure form into the vitreous cavity, they will expand due to the infusion of nitrogen and other blood gases into the gas pocket. A pure SF_6 gas bubble injected into the vitreous cavity will expand approximately 2.5 times its injection volume. A pure C_3F_8 gas bubble will expand approximately 4 times its injected volume. Both gases expand at approximately the same rate. There is risk of ocular hypertension and vascular occlusion when pure gases are used during vitreous surgery. Because of the risk of ocular hypertension, we prefer to use "nonexpansile" gases at surgery. For use in vitreous surgery, 20% SF_6 and 14% PFP are essentially nonexpansile and safe.

Intraocular gases are injected at the end of the procedure following reattachment of the retina with a fluid-air exchange. We inject the gas by the method of air-gas exchange. At the completion of the procedure, the two instrument sclerotomy sites are completely closed. Approximately 40 cc of the selected gas mixture are flushed through the air-filled eye through the infusion port and vented by a 27-gauge needle inserted through the pars plana into the vitreous cavity. The needle is attached to a tuberculin syringe from which the plunger has been removed to form a "chimney" to allow the egress of the flushed gas. The eye may need to be reformed with the gas mixture to a normal intraocular pressure following removal of the infusion port and closure of the last sclerotomy site.

The major risk of the use of intraocular gas is ocular hypertension. By using a nonexpansile concentration of the gas, the risk of ocular hypertension is markedly decreased. Intraocular pressure and light perception can be checked 2–4 hours after surgery since the intraocular pressure of an expansile bubble tends to peak at approximately this time. We give topical ocular antihypertensive medications at the conclusion of surgery. Some surgeons also use oral acetazolamide through the first postoperative night. Special attention is given to high risk eyes, including eyes with pre-existing glaucoma, hyperopic eyes, eyes with scleral buckle, and eyes with extensive laser panretinal photocoagulation at surgery. It is important to position the patient prone or on one side to prevent pupillary block by the gas bubble. There is risk of cataract formation if the gas bubble stays in prolonged contact with the lens of the phakic eye.

Silicone Oil

Silicone oil is useful in the treatment of proliferative vitreoretinopathy, giant retinal tears, some eyes of diabetics with complicated retinal detachments or with severe anterior segment neovascularization. The silicone study showed no significant difference between C_3F_8 gas and silicone oil in management of eyes with PVR. Eyes managed with gas had a slightly higher retinal reattachment rate than eyes managed with oil in eyes that had not had a previous vitrectomy (group 1 eyes). However there was no difference in the percent of eyes with visual acuity of 5/200 or better and there was no difference in either retinal reattachment rate or visual acuity in eyes that had had a previous vitrectomy with gas (group 2 eyes). Hypotony, IOP $\leq$5 mm Hg was more common in gas eyes than oil eyes, whether the retina was attached or not and whether the eye had had a previous vitrectomy with gas or not. Eyes with large retinotomies did better with oil than gas. Longer tamponade provided by C_3F_8 gas or silicone oil was preferable to the shorter tamponade provided by SF_6 gas. Silicone oil was removed from most eyes with attached retinas, normal intraocular pressures, clear corneas, and better visual acuities. Conversely, silicone oil was less commonly removed from eyes with detached retinas, poorer visual acuities, corneal abnormalities, and hypotony. Eyes managed with silicone oil that had the silicone oil removed had better outcomes than eyes with oil retained or eyes managed with gas. Silicone oil is preferred over gas in patients unable to maintain a prone position after surgery and for patients that need to fly in an airplane or travel to a higher altitude. Gas may be preferred in eyes with residual hemorrhage, eyes without an adequate iris diaphragm, and eyes with retinal breaks on the posterior slope of very high scleral buckles. In the latter instance, because the silicone oil bubble might not conform to the shape of the high scleral buckle, the retinal breaks might not be adequately closed.

In diabetic retinopathy, silicone oil may be useful in eyes with severe anterior segment neovascular complications, including neovascular glaucoma and anterior hyaloidal fibrovascular proliferation. High vascular endothelial growth factor levels have been documented in the anterior chamber of eyes with neovascularization of the iris. The silicone oil may block the circulation of such growth factors into the anterior segment. In addition, oil may be useful in some eyes of diabetics with complicated retinal detachments requiring extensive retinotomies. These eyes are often very ischemic, so the visual prognosis is poor, but such eyes can sometimes be stabilized with silicone oil.

Silicone oil may be helpful in eyes with giant tears or giant retinotomies. Most giant retinal tears are repaired with vitrectomy and unfolding of the flap of the giant tear with PFCL. When the PFCL is removed and exchanged for air, the edge of the giant tear can "slip" (slide posteriorly), creating a retinal fold posterior to the tear. This slippage is produced by fluid collection behind the anterior retina that may not be fully reattached by the PFCL. As the air goes into the eye, it can force the fluid posteriorly, creating the slippage and the fold. Directly exchanging the PFCL for silicone oil will usually prevent slippage of the flap. Because the buoyancy of the silicone oil is less than that of air, there is less force applied to the retina as the silicone oil is infused, and there is less tendency to force subretinal fluid posteriorly. Silicone oil may be advantageous if there is proliferation of membranes that apply traction to the retina following giant tear repair. The silicone oil tends to localize recurrent retinal detachment due to proliferative membranes and these eyes can sometimes be managed with a relatively simple membrane peeling procedure under silicone oil or after silicone oil removal. Eyes managed with gas are more likely to totally redetach if proliferative membranes form, especially if a retinal break is present.

Silicone oil is injected using one of two techniques. In the most commonly used technique, the retina is reattached with a fluid-air exchange or, alternatively, with PFCL. We usually apply laser treatment under PFCL or air, prior to silicone oil infusion. If PFCL is used, the PFCL is exchanged for air. The silicone oil is infused into the air-filled eye. In this method, the silicone oil is pumped into the eye to fill the vitreous cavity to the level of the iris diaphragm. The anterior chamber is left filled with fluid or air. The second method is by PFCL-silicone oil exchange. As the silicone oil is pumped into the eye with a silicone pump, the PFCL is passively evacuated with a fluted needle with backflush capability. Perfluorocarbon liquid-silicone oil exchange is more easily done with 1000-centistoke silicone oil than with 5000-centistoke silicone oil. Any subretinal fluid beneath the peripheral retina can be removed with a backflush brush held at any anterior retinal breaks. The backflush capability of the needle allows easy release of the retina. We most commonly use PFCL-silicone oil exchange when there is a giant retinal tear or retinotomy more than 270 degrees in circumference, when there is a risk of posterior slippage of the flap. This is also a useful technique if a silicone IOL is present. With air or gas in the vitreous cavity, there is condensation on the posterior surface of the silicone IOL that obscures the view of the vitreous cavity. While the view is better when silicone oil is used, the silicone oil adheres to the IOL and obscures the view if the silicone oil is removed. The IOL must be removed if the silicone oil is removed.

There are several potential complications of silicone oil. The major complication is corneal damage, which occurs when silicone oil is in contact with the endothelium. Retrocorneal membranes form and band keratopathy is common. Corneal contact by the silicone oil can be prevented in the aphakic eye by creating an inferior iridectomy. When silicone oil remains in contact with the lens, a feathery posterior subcapsular cataract is produced.

With prolonged silicone oil-lens contact, a permanent cataract will form in all cases. Therefore, if silicone oil is used in phakic eyes, it should be removed as soon as possible (usually within 4–6 weeks).

Glaucoma can result from emulsification of the silicone oil. Small bubbles can pass into the anterior chamber and obstruct the trabecular meshwork. Emulsification is most commonly seen when there is substantial movement of the silicone oil associated with a loose iris diaphragm. Emulsification is probably also more common with mixed silicone oils of various molecular weights and densities. Use of purified silicone oil reduces the incidence of this complication. Emulsification is more common with 1000-centistoke silicone oil than with the 5000-centistoke variety. If emulsification is seen, the silicone oil should probably be removed because of the risk of glaucoma.

Proliferation of fibrous tissue that is sometimes seen with silicone oil is most commonly associated with large retinotomies or retinectomies and is accentuated by the presence of preretinal blood. If recurrent membranes are seen following silicone oil injection, the membranes should be removed and the silicone oil evacuated from the eye, if possible.

Giant Retinal Tears

Giant retinal tears are retinal tears greater than 90 degrees in circumference. Giant retinal tears are unique among retinal detachments because the flap of the retina posterior to the giant tear may fold posteriorly and may be difficult to return to its normal position. Giant tears are usually repaired surgically with vitreous surgery. The goals of the surgery are to relieve retinal traction, unfold the flap of the giant tear if necessary, and create a retinal adhesion between the torn retina and the underlying retinal pigment epithelium (RPE), usually with laser photocoagulation. It may be necessary to remove epiretinal or subretinal membranes and place a scleral buckle.

Surgical Technique

If PVR is present, we remove the crystalline lens, even if clear. For giant tears without PVR, we usually retain the lens if the tear is less than 180 degrees, but remove the lens in larger giant tears. If the lens is retained we usually place a scleral buckle, because there may be residual anterior vitreous that may be associated with postoperative anterior traction. However, if the lens is removed and there is no significant PVR, it may be possible to avoid a scleral buckle because it is possible to remove most of the anterior vitreous, thus avoiding anterior traction. We remove the vitreous gel and carefully remove anterior vitreous. A wide-angle viewing system is helpful for the anterior portion of the vitrectomy, and scleral depression will help with anterior vitreous removal. If there is PVR present,

we then remove epiretinal membranes starting at the posterior pole, progressing anteriorly. After we remove posterior membranes, PFCL can be injected to stabilize the posterior retina as anterior membranes are removed (Figure 8-28A). We usually excise nonfunctional retina anterior to the giant tear, and make sure all vitreous and membranes are removed at the ends of the giant tear. Following removal of all membranes if present, the PFCL can be injected to unfold and flatten the flap of the giant tear (Figure 8-31A). If the flap is mobile, the PFCL can be injected until the level is anterior to the level of the tear (Figure 8-31B). If the edge is folded,

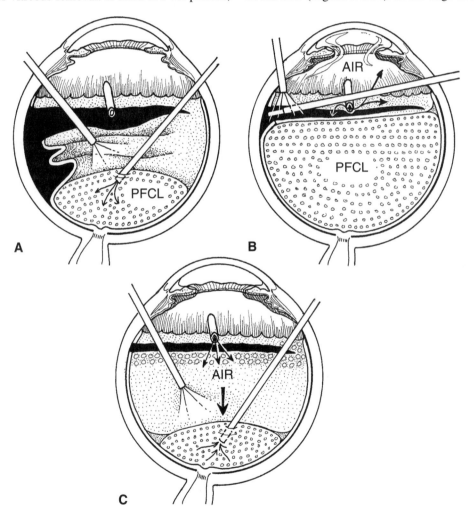

Figure 8-31. Management of giant retinal tear or retinotomy with PFCL. **A,** Retina reattached from posteriorly to anteriorly with PFCL. This unfolds flap of giant tear. **B,** After retina attached, fluid-air exchange. "Drying" edge of giant tear by aspirating fluid from beneath anterior edge of tear will prevent posterior slippage of flap of tear. **C,** Continuation of fluid-air exchange without posterior slippage of edge of tear. Adapted from Abrams GW, Gentile RC. Vitrectomy. In: Guyer DR, Yannuzzi LA, Chang S, Shields JA, Green WR, eds. *Retina-Vitreous-Macula*. Vol. 2. Philadelphia: W.B. Saunders; 1999:1309.

PFCL should remain posterior to the folded edge of the retina. The anterior folds can usually be unfolded with the illuminated pick and forceps. However, in the event that the edge is so folded and fixed that it cannot be completely freed, the folded edge should be excised with the vitreous cutter. We apply endodiathermy to the area to be excised to prevent bleeding. After the edge is attached with PFCL, we apply two or three rows of laser endophotocoagulation to the edge of the tear. We also treat the untorn anterior retina with two or three rows of laser in a scatter pattern. A scleral buckle is more likely needed for smaller giant tears than larger tears. The scleral buckle is used to support the ends of the giant tear and the untorn retina. If there is no PVR and a lensectomy has been done, it may be possible to remove enough vitreous to release all traction on the retina. For giant tears less than 270 degrees, if a lensectomy is not done, we usually place a scleral buckle. A scatter pattern of endolaser photocoagulation is placed on the retina supported by the scleral buckle. If a scleral buckle is anticipated, we prefer to preplace the mattress sutures in the sclera prior to the vitrectomy as suture placement is easier and safer at that time. We usually use an encircling band, 3.5–4.0 mm wide, but wait until the vitrectomy is complete and the retina is attached before placing the buckle around the eye. A low buckle is usually desirable to prevent posterior slippage of the retina and radial folds.

We remove the PFCL with a PFCL-air (Figure 8-31C) or PFCL-silicone oil exchange. If a PFCL-air exchange is done, it is important to "dry" the edge of the giant tear in the initial portion of the exchange as mentioned previously (see Figure 8-31B). If silicone oil is to be used in the aphakic eye, we create an inferior iridectomy prior to removing the PFCL. The decision to use silicone oil or gas depends on a number of factors, including surgeon preference. We mentioned indications for silicone oil when discussing the silicone study previously. Those indications are similar for giant tears. Eyes with giant tears and PVR generally do better with silicone oil than gas; however, those without PVR probably do equally well with oil or gas. Silicone oil requires less strict prone positioning and may prevent total retinal detachment if membranes proliferate postoperatively. Patients are able to travel to high altitudes and fly with silicone oil present, but not with gas. Silicone oil must be removed, while gas is absorbed spontaneously. We usually remove silicone oil within 6 weeks to 3 months following surgery.

Membrane Removal in Diabetic Retinopathy

Clinical Appearance and Indications

Fibrovascular proliferation in diabetic retinopathy originates from focal epicenters on blood vessels of the optic nerve head and the retina. Fibrovascular tissue grows as a sheet in the potential space between the retina and the vitreous. Contraction of the fibrovascular tissue may cause contraction of the vitreous that may exert traction on the new vessels, causing hemorrhage. Hemorrhage usually occurs from tearing of the blood vessels within the membrane. Traction retinal detachment may occur and retinal breaks can occur adjacent to areas of traction, causing a traction-rhegmatogenous retinal detachment. The goal of diabetic vitrectomy is to clear the media (remove hemorrhage) and to release vitreoretinal traction. There are two major elements to the traction in diabetic retinopathy. The first is AP traction from contraction of the vitreous with traction transmitted from the vitreous base peripherally to the area of the fibrovascular membranes posteriorly where vitreoretinal adhesion is present. The second form is tangential traction, which is primarily posteriorly in areas of posterior fibrovascular membranes. Posterior tangential traction is due to contraction of fibrovascular membranes between the epicenters of fibrovascular proliferation. The traction is transmitted via the fibrovascular membranes and the partially detached posterior hyaloid.

Surgical Technique

We separate the posterior hyaloid and the associated fibrovascular tissue as a single unit from the retinal surface whenever possible, using a technique called "en bloc" excision of the diabetic membranes and the associated posterior hyaloid. We perform an initial partial vitrectomy to remove the posterior hyaloid adjacent to the fibrovascular tissue (Figure 8-32). We usually remove the posterior hyaloid temporal to the posterior pole, as well as the vitreous posterior to the temporal sclerotomy site where

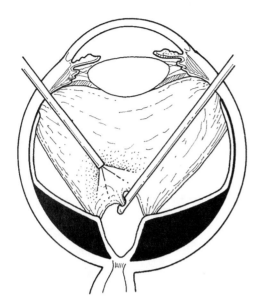

Figure 8-32. Vitrectomy for diabetic retinopathy. Excision of vitreous around posterior vitreoretinal adhesions. Adapted from Lewis JM, Abrams GW, Werner JC. Management of complicated retinal detachment. In: Albert DM, ed. *Ophthalmic Surgery: Principles and Techniques.* Vol. 1. Malden, MA: Blackwell Science; 1999:1309.

the scissors are placed in the eye. In some eyes the posterior hyaloid is only minimally separated from the retina and the posterior hyaloid is opened in the area of separation. Any blood is removed from the subhyaloid space through the limited opening. We prefer to use the "tissue manipulator" (see Figure 8-6), a multifunctional instrument with endoillumi-

nation, endodiathermy, and a blunt 30-gauge cannula on the end for aspiration to hold the tissue during dissection and to displace blood from the retinal surface so the source of hemorrhage can be identified and treated with endodiathermy. For excision of membranes from the retina, we use the MPC scissors (Alcon Laboratories, Fort Worth), or alternatively, the horizontally cutting Sutherland scissors. The hyaloid is initially separated from the epicenters using an illuminated membrane pick and/or the closed tips of the scissors. The posterior hyaloid between the epicenters will strip cleanly from the retina, exposing the epicenters. The epicenters are then cut parallel to, and flush with the retinal surface (Figure 8-33A). We elevate the membrane during cutting with the aspiration function of the tissue manipulator. This allows bimanual removal of the membranes and enhances visualization of the epicenter of the membrane. Alternatively, illuminated forceps or picks can be used to elevate membranes. The membranes separate from the retina as the epicenters are cut, better exposing the remaining epicenters of proliferation. Each is individually cut as it is exposed to release the fibrovascular membrane from the retinal surface. Minor bleeding sometimes occurs from the vessels severed at the epicenters, but this will usually stop spontaneously. Raising the pressure in the eye by raising the infusion bottles for a short period of time will control most persistent hemorrhage. Diathermy is applied to any persistent bleeding points on the retinal surface. Light direct pressure

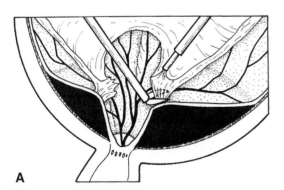

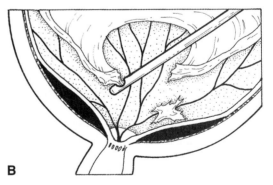

A **B**

Figure 8-33. Vitrectomy for diabetic retinopathy. **A,** Membrane and attached vitreous elevated with tissue manipulator as membrane is excised with scissors parallel with the retinal surface. **B,** Following separation of vitreous, vitreous removed with vitreous cutter. Adapted from Lewis JM, Abrams GW, Werner JC. Management of complicated retinal detachment. In: Albert DM, ed. *Ophthalmic Surgery: Principles and Techniques.* Vol. 1. Malden, MA: Blackwell Science; 1999:1309.

can also be applied with the edge of the vitrectomy instrument if other techniques are ineffective. After the fibrovascular membrane is separated from the retina, any remaining posterior hyaloid attached to the retina is stripped free to the far periphery. The fibrovascular membranes and the vitreous are then excised using the vitreous cutting instrument (Figure 8-33B). We remove remaining fibrovascular tissue on the retina surface by lifting the tissue with the tissue manipulator and cutting with the scissors (Figure 8-34).

We have found complete excision of diabetic membranes to be superior to membrane sectioning techniques. There is less hemorrhage when the epicenters are excised compared to cutting across (sectioning) the fibrovascular membranes. There is also less chance of occult retinal breaks being hidden by residual fibrous tissue left behind with membrane sectioning techniques. We believe that there is less postoperative hemorrhage when membranes are excised rather than sectioned as well as less risk of membrane reproliferation.

Other Techniques

A number of vitrectomy procedures have been introduced for macular diseases. Macular holes can now be treated with vitrectomy (see Chapter 9). Other macular techniques have been developed for subfoveal choroidal neovascular membrane removal and foveal translocation. The indications for surgical removal of subfoveal choroidal neovascular membranes have not been well defined. Early reports indicate a likely benefit for patients with ocular histoplasmosis syndrome (OHS), but less so for other causes of subretinal neovascularization. The indications and outcomes of surgery for subfoveal choroidal neovascular membranes due to OHS and age-related macular degeneration (ARMD) are being investigated in the subretinal surgery trial (SST), a multicenter, randomized, controlled clinical trial sponsored by the National Eye Institute. In addition, the SST is comparing surgical evacuation of large subretinal hemorrhages associated with ARMD with no surgery.

Surgical Technique: Subfoveal Neovascular Membrane Removal

Following vitrectomy, we separate the posterior cortical vitreous from the retina. Using a 36–40-gauge sharp spatula, a small retinotomy is made adjacent to the subfoveal choroidal neovascular membrane. If no subretinal fluid is present, we inject balanced saline solution with a microcannula through the retinotomy into the subretinal space to elevate the retina over the subretinal neovascular membrane. If subretinal fluid is already present, fluid injection is not necessary. The infusion bottle is raised to elevate the intraocular pressure to temporarily cause stasis of blood flow. We then place a blunt spatula through the retinotomy into the subretinal space and we make an attempt to separate the neovascular complex from the surrounding tissue. This is particularly important if the membrane is adherent to retinal pigment epithelium (RPE), which can rip during removal of the membrane and cause a large area of RPE loss. The tip of a subretinal forceps is then placed through the retinotomy to grasp the subretinal neovascular membrane and gently elevate it and separate it from its underlying vascular attachment. There may be a single, small vascular frond attached to the choroidal side of the membrane that will separate when the membrane is slowly withdrawn. Sometimes, however, the base of the membrane can be broad and adherent, causing a significant RPE defect when the membrane and adhering RPE are removed. We maintain high intraocular pressure for approximately 3 minutes

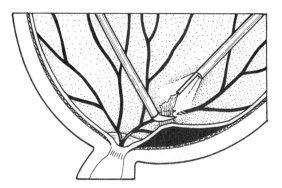

Figure 8-34. Excision of isolated vitreoretinal membrane. Membrane elevated with tissue manipulator and excised with scissors parallel to retinal surface. Adapted from Lewis JM, Abrams GW, Werner JC. Management of complicated retinal detachment. In: Albert DM, ed. *Ophthalmic Surgery: Principles and Techniques.* Vol. 1. Malden, MA: Blackwell Science; 1999:1309.

and then slowly lower the IOP until the IOP is normalized. If hemorrhage reoccurs, we once more elevate the IOP for 3–5 minutes, then slowly lower the IOP. After hemostasis is confirmed, we inspect the peripheral retina for retinal breaks; if none are present, we proceed to a fluid-air exchange. We subtotally fill the vitreous cavity with air, then close as described above. Prone positioning is enforced for the first 24 hours postoperatively.

Retinal Translocation with 360-Degree Retinotomy

Retinal or foveal translocation surgery may be useful for selected subfoveal choroidal neovascular membranes. The goal of both techniques is to move the fovea from abnormal RPE to a new position over more normal RPE. Since these are new techniques, reports are limited and the indications and outcomes are still unclear. Retinal translocation with 360-degree retinotomy is used for large subfoveal choroidal neovascular membranes and is more difficult than the limited foveal translocation procedure. In retinal translocation, the vitreous is separated from the retina and the retina is totally detached by injecting BSS transretinally with a 39- or 40-gauge cannula. It may be necessary to inject through more than one retinotomy to completely detach the retina. After the retina is detached, it is quite bullous; then a 360-degree retinotomy is made as far peripherally as possible. The retinotomy is best made while viewing through a noncontact wide-angle viewing system. The retina is rotated to the desired position around the optic nerve, then reattached with PFCL. The retinotomy is treated with two or three rows of laser endophotocoagulation. Silicone oil is infused into the eye during fluid-silicone oil exchange and the eye is left filled with silicone oil.

It is important to shave the peripheral vitreous flush with the vitreous base. This is difficult in the phakic eye, so the lens is removed in most cases. Some surgeons place a posterior chamber IOL at the time of vitrectomy, while others will place the IOL during a second surgery. Because there may be rotation of 25–50 degrees, severe torsional diplopia may result. It may be necessary to rotate the eye with torsional muscle surgery. Some surgeons do the muscle surgery at the same sitting as the retinal translocation surgery.

Limited Foveal Translocation

Limited foveal translocation is used for smaller subfoveal choroidal neovascular membranes. Prior to vitrectomy, we preplace five or six mattress sutures so as to cause superotemporal circumferential, equatorial imbrication of the sclera over an area of approximately 120 degrees, when the sutures are tightened following vitrectomy. One suture is placed just nasal to the superior rectus muscle, four sutures are placed in the superotemporal quadrant, and one suture is placed just inferior to the lateral rectus muscle. During the vitrectomy procedure, the vitreous is separated from the retina, then the retina is detached by injecting BSS transretinally with a 40-gauge cannula. We limit the artificial retinal detachment to the temporal 180 degrees plus part of the adjacent superonasal retina. It is important to detach the macula, as well as the peripheral retina. It may be useful to do a partial fluid-air exchange to force bullous retina posteriorly to aid in macular detachment. With the retina detached and air filling the anterior portion of the vitreous cavity, we tie the imbrication sutures. We then do additional fluid-air exchange to fill approximately 50–60% of the vitreous cavity with air. No subretinal fluid is drained.

Postoperatively, the patient is positioned upright to move the retina inferiorly. The limited foveal translocation technique typically moves the fovea from 200–1300 µ, much less than can be attained with the retinal translocation with 360-degree retinotomy technique. It may be necessary to treat the choroidal neovascular membrane with laser photocoagulation postoperatively. Patients may experience transient torsional diplopia, but this usually resolves in a matter of months.

Both translocation techniques can be complicated by retinal detachment and/or PVR. Randomized, controlled clinical trials are needed to determine the value of these procedures.

Other Indications for Vitrectomy

There are other important indications for vitrectomy and vitrectomy procedures that are beyond the scope of this chapter. Vitrectomy removal or repositioning of a dislocated IOL is an important indication. Bacterial or fungal, exogenous or endogenous endophthalmitis, retinopathy of prematurity, and severe

CMV retinitis each may require specialized vitrectomy equipment and techniques.

Intraoperative Complications of Vitrectomy

Vitreous surgery is accompanied by many potential complications, some new and unique to vitreous surgery and others common to other intraocular procedures. Complications are more common in severely diseased eyes. Intraoperative complications are classified as entrance-site complications, lens complications, acute ocular hypertension, hemorrhages, and retinal tears and detachment. Corneal complications, postoperative glaucoma, endophthalmitis, and sympathetic ophthalmia will be discussed in Chapter 10. The major entrance-site complications are uveal infusion and subretinal infusion. If the infusion port fails to perforate the pars plana pigmented or nonpigmented epithelium, infusion fluids feed into the suprachoroidal space (Figure 8-35) or the subretinal space. Uveal or subretinal infusion is best prevented by always ascertaining that the tip of the infusion port has perforated the pars plana epithelium prior to turning on the infusion. Treatment involves removing the infusion port and then infusing fluid into the vitreous cavity through the vitrectomy instrument or a needle (Figure 8-36). Suprachoroidal fluid escapes through the now open sclerotomy site.

Peripheral retinal dialysis can occur when instruments placed through the sclerotomy site exert traction on the peripheral vitreous (Figure 8-37). Although the incidence of peripheral dialysis is low when small-gauge instruments are used,

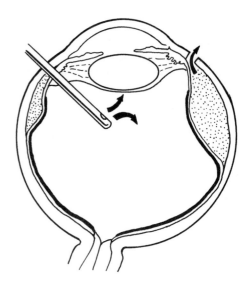

Figure 8-36. Drainage of choroidal infusion. Infusion port removed to allow drainage of suprachoroidal fluid. Fluid infused into vitreous cavity through vitreous cutter. Alternatively, fluid can be injected through needle.

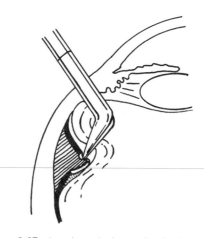

Figure 8-37. Anterior retinal tear related to insertion of scissors though sclerotomy. Tear caused by traction on vitreous base by scissors tip.

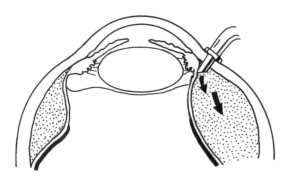

Figure 8-35. Choroidal infusion caused by incomplete penetration of pars plana epithelium by infusion port.

peripheral tears still occur. The use of entrance-site trocars and cannulas probably reduces the incidence of entrance-site dialysis.

Vitreous or retina can incarcerate in the sclerotomy site. Some vitreous is probably incarcerated in the sclerotomy site at the end of surgery in most cases. This can, on occasion, lead to intraocular fibrous proliferation and retinal traction or late tears of the retina due to traction. It is helpful to pay attention to reducing the amount of vitreous incarceration in the wounds by lowering the infusion pressure before removing instruments. Vitreous should be removed from the lips of the sclerotomy sites prior to closure using the vitreous cutter and/or dry cellulose sponges and small scissors. Retinal incarceration can occur in the sclerotomy in an eye with a bullous retinal detachment and is best avoided by turning off the infusion before removing instruments. A viscoelastic injection at the sclerotomy site or the use of a smooth instrument may dislodge incarcerated retina from the sclerotomy site. As an alternative, the incarcerated retina can be removed from the sclerotomy site internally with forceps or a suction needle (silicone tip) placed into the eye through another sclerotomy site. PFCL injected over the posterior retina will sometimes disengage retina from the sclerotomy site.

Corneal erosions are most common in diabetics and appear to be less of a problem now than in earlier reports. Corneal epithelium should be protected preoperatively by using as little phenylephrine as possible and intraoperatively by protecting the cornea from drying and trauma. Improved infusion solutions used during surgery have probably helped to reduce the incidence of severe cornea problems following vitrectomy. Corneal complications include recurrent erosions, (usually most severe in diabetic eyes), filamentary keratitis, and bullous keratopathy. Postoperative erosions are treated with patching and emollients. Persistent erosions can be treated with bandage contact lenses.

Lens damage can result from direct trauma to the lens. This usually occurs during removal of peripheral vitreous when an instrument comes in contact with the lens. Improvements in infusion solutions have reduced the incidence of intraoperative lens opacification. The use of glucose-fortified BSS plus infusion has reduced the incidence of cataract in diabetics.

The cornea can be damaged and there can be hemorrhage and iridodialysis during pars plana ultrasound lensectomy. These complications are best prevented by keeping ultrasound fragmentation to a minimum and using gentle, controlled suction when near the iris.

Intraoperative acute ocular hypertension may produce visually significant problems by occluding choroidal and/or retinal vasculature. During surgery the surgeon must be aware of the intraocular pressure. The infusion bottle should not be raised to a high level for a prolonged period of time. Postoperative glaucoma may result from hemorrhage, inflammation, choroidal edema, orbital hemorrhage, pupillary block mechanisms, expansile gases, or neovascular glaucoma. This will be considered in Chapter 10.

Intraoperative or postoperative hemorrhage may occur. Hemorrhage during vitrectomy may arise from iris or angle vessels, retinal vessels, retinal neovascularization, or choroidal vessels. Hemorrhage is more likely to occur in a hypotonous eye than when the intraocular pressure is elevated, because the pressure gradient between the vascular system and the eye is greater during hypotony. Hemorrhage can initially be controlled by increasing the intraocular pressure by raising the infusion bottle. The source of hemorrhage should be identified and treated with bipolar endodiathermy. Light direct pressure from the rounded edge of the vitrectomy instrument can be effective. Severe uncontrolled hemorrhage may be managed with the infusion of intraocular thrombin (100-cc solution with a concentration of 100 units per cc). Postoperative hemorrhage may be the result of residual hemorrhage from surgery, retained blood within the vitreous, or continued hemorrhage from bleeding sites. Minor hemorrhage will usually clear spontaneously, but denser hemorrhage may need to be removed. Hemorrhage can sometimes be removed with a postoperative fluid-air exchange or may sometimes require a vitreous washout procedure.

Retinal tears and retinal detachment may occur during vitrectomy or during membrane removal procedures. Posterior breaks, if not under traction, can be managed with air or gas injection techniques. Peripheral breaks do not require a scleral buckle if all traction is relieved. If persistent traction is present, an encircling scleral buckle is necessary. In most cases of retinal detachment associated with vitrectomy, a fluid-gas exchange is performed or PFCL is injected to reattach the retina. Some form of intraocular tamponade is necessary when the retina is detached following vitrectomy. Tamponade with air, gas, or silicone oil is used for retinal detachments associated with vitrectomy. Retinal breaks are treated with cryopexy or laser endophotocoagulation.

Suggested Reading

Aaberg TM. Management of anterior and posterior proliferative vitreoretinopathy. XLV Edward Jackson Memorial Lecture. *Am J Ophthalmol* 1988;106:519.

Abrams GW, Azen SP, McCuen BW II, et al. Vitrectomy with silicone oil or long-acting gas in eyes with severe proliferative vitreoretinopathy: results of additional and long-term follow-up (Silicone Study Report 11). *Arch Ophthalmol* 1997;115:335–344.

Abrams GW, Gentile RC. Vitrectomy. In: Guyer DR, Yannuzzi LA, Chang S, Shields JA, Green WR, eds. *Retina-Vitreous-Macula*. Vol. 2. Philadelphia: Saunders; 1999:1298–1319.

Abrams GW, Nanda S. Retinotomies and retinectomies. In: Ryan SF, ed. *Retina*. Vol. 3. 3rd ed. St. Louis: Mosby; 2000.

Chang S. Low viscosity liquid fluorochemicals in vitreous surgery. *Am J Ophthalmol* 1987;103:38.

Chang S, Lincoff H, Coleman DJ, Fuchs W, Farber ME. Perfluorocarbon gases in vitreous surgery. *Ophthalmology* 1985;92:651.

Eliott D, Abrams GW. Vitrectomy for diabetic retinopathy. In: Ryan SF, ed. *Retina*. Vol. 3. 3rd ed. St. Louis: Mosby; 2000.

Lewis JM, Abrams GW, Werner JC. Management of complicated retinal detachment. In: Albert DM, ed. *Ophthalmic Surgery: Principles and Practice*. Vol. 1. Malden, MA: Blackwell Science; 1999:531–566.

Silicone Study Group. Vitrectomy with silicone oil or perfluoropropane gas in eyes with severe proliferative vitreoretinopathy: results of a randomized clinical trial (Silicone Study Report 2). *Arch Ophthalmol* 1992;110:780–792.

Zivojnovic R. *Silicone Oil in Vitreoretinal Surgery*. Dordrecht: Martinus Nijhoff; 1987.

9

Macular Hole Surgery

Lawrence S. Morse, Robert T. Wendel, and Peter T. Yip

Goals of Macular Hole Surgery

The surgical goal for macular hole surgery is to facilitate anatomic closure of the macular hole. As first reported by Kelly and Wendel in 1991,[1] this is achieved by the use of vitrectomy techniques to relieve anterior-posterior and/or tangential traction and the use of retinal tamponade to facilitate reapproximation of the retina to the retinal pigment epithelium (RPE). The traction is relieved by identification and removal of the cortical and posterior hyaloidal vitreous, and removal of tangential traction caused by epiretinal membranes (ERM) and/or the internal limiting membrane (ILM) around the hole. Tamponade is provided by injection of a long-acting gas, sulfur hexafluoride (SF6) or perfluoropropane (C3F8), and strict face-down positioning for 1–2 weeks.

Indications

The major indications for macular hole surgery are listed in Table 9-1. Our indications for surgical intervention are vision loss and the presence of a full-thickness retinal break. Clinically, we have found very little use in dwelling on whether a macular hole is classified as stage 2, stage 3, or stage 4 (Table 9-2, Gass classification). Because our observations that good preoperative vision, short duration, and small holes are favorable predictors for both anatomic and visual success and because the

natural history is unfavorable, we are intervening earlier than in the past.[2]

Vitreous surgery for impending macular holes (stage 1) is not considered routinely for the following reasons: (1) difficulty in making the correct diagnosis of impending macular holes, (2) unproven therapeutic benefit, (3) cost and complications of surgery, (4) spontaneous recovery in many patients, and (5) good anatomic and functional results after macular hole surgery for early full-thickness macular holes.[3]

The same techniques used for an idiopathic macular hole can be applied to macular holes of other etiologies. Vision loss secondary to macular hole associated with rhegmatogenous retinal detachment has been successfully treated with macular hole surgery (MHS). Likewise, macular holes after pneumatic retinopexy have been managed successfully with MHS.

Table 9-1. Indication for Macular Hole Surgery

Vision loss and presence of a full-thickness retinal break secondary to:
 a. Idiopathic macular holes
 b. Macular holes associated with rhegmatogenous retinal detachment
 c. Macular holes after pneumatic retinopexy
 d. Traumatic macular holes
 e. Macular hole after macular pucker surgery
 f. Macular holes associated with macular degeneration, high myopia, adult vitelliform dystrophy, Best's disease, retinitis pigmentosa, diabetic retinopathy, and peripheral telangiectasia

Table 9-2. Gass Classification of Macular Holes

Stages	Clinical Appearance	Fluorescein Angiography
1a, 1b	A yellow spot, 100–200 μ in diameter (1a), or yellow ring, 200–300 μ in diameter (1b) at the fovea	Faint hyperfluorescence or no abnormality
2	Full-thickness defect/dehiscence	Round area of window defect or normal
3	Full-thickness defect ≥400 μ in diameter, a surrounding cuff of edema and fluid, with or without pseudo-operculum	Window defect corresponding to the hole
4	Further development of a complete posterior vitreous detachment, with anterior displacement of the pseudo-operculum	Window defect corresponding to the hole

Traumatic macular holes frequently are associated with other ocular injuries, including RPE disruption and choroidal rupture. The patients usually are young men. Although most cases arise from penetrating or blunt trauma; other injuries, such as industrial laser burns, may result in a traumatic macular hole. Experience has shown traumatic macular holes can also be repaired with MHS. Rubin and colleagues[4] reported on 12 cases of MHS for traumatic macular holes. They were able to close 92% of the holes with one or more operations and achieved 20/40 or better vision in 50% of their cases.

Successful MHS has also been performed on eyes that developed holes after macular pucker surgery, and on holes associated with macular degeneration, high myopia, adult vitelliform dystrophy, Best's disease, retinitis pigmentosa, diabetic retinopathy, and peripheral telangiectasia.[5]

Prognostic Factors

Favorable prognostic factors are listed in Table 9-3. Eyes with earlier-stage holes, shorter macular hole duration, and better preoperative visual acuity have a better prognosis for anatomic and visual success (Figure 9-1).[6] Kelly and Wendel[1] reported that anatomic success rate in holes of ≤ 6 months was 80%, for 6–24 months' duration was 74%, and for >24 months was 22%. Postoperative visual success rates declined with increasing duration of

Table 9-3. Favorable Prognostic Factors

- Preoperative VA ≥20/100
- Duration of symptoms ≤1 year
- Small size of macular hole ≤450 μ
- Stage 2 or 3 macular hole

symptoms (Figure 9-2). Ryan and Gilbert[7] reported a 95% anatomic success rate in early-stage holes (stage 2) versus 60% in late-stage holes (stages 3 and 4). The size of the macular hole may be the most important physical characteristic, as the size probably is related to duration, stage, and visual acuity.[6]

Case Selection

Today, most eyes with macular holes are candidates for surgery. Relative contraindications include patients unable to maintain prone positioning, some cases of traumatic macular hole with additional ocular injuries, and long-standing or asymptomatic macular holes. If the fellow eye is normal, conservative management can be discussed with the patient. Just as obtaining consent is advised before surgery, the medical record should document clearly that MHS was discussed, as were the reasons for a conservative approach. We are aware of one case of legal action brought against a physician that alleged delayed treatment of a macular hole. Informed consent should include discussion of MHS complications that may arise intraoperatively as well as during the early and late postoperative periods.

Preoperative Evaluation

Many conditions mimic a macular hole for which either no treatment or different surgical maneuvers are needed. These conditions include epiretinal membrane, geographic atrophy of the RPE and overlying retina, cystoid macular edema, lamellar macular holes, subfoveal choroidal neovascularization with a foveal cyst and intraretinal edema, and vitreomacular traction with a cystic fovea.[8] Careful

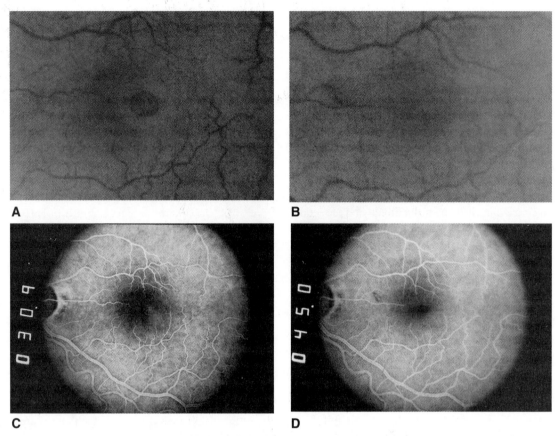

Figure 9-1. **A,** Preoperative photograph of a patient with a macular hole and 20/100 vision. **B,** Postoperative photograph of the same patient showing a "closed" macular hole. Vision improved to 20/50. **C,** Preoperative fluorescein angiogram of the same patient showing a central hyperfluorescent window defect. **D,** Postoperative fluorescein angiogram of the same patient showing partial resolution of a central hyperfluorescent window defect.

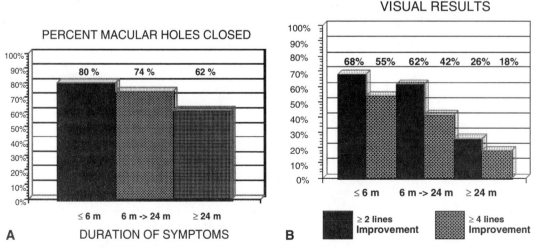

Figure 9-2. **A,** Anatomic success is inversely related to duration of symptoms. Eighty percent of eyes symptomatic for 6 months or less were anatomically successful, 74% if symptomatic for 6 months to 2 years, and 61% of those symptomatic for 2 years or more. **B,** Visual success is inversely related to duration of symptoms. Sixty-eight percent of eyes symptomatic for 6 months or less improved by two lines or more, whereas only 26% of eyes symptomatic for 2 years or more improved.

clinical examination is needed to differentiate macular holes from the other pseudohole conditions.

The various stages of macular holes are described according to the Gass classification (see Table 9-2). Biomicroscopy is the most important technique used to clinically evaluate macular holes. Fundus fluorescein angiography is also frequently used and may demonstrate an RPE window defect corresponding to the macular hole. In addition to fluorescein angiography, other ancillary tests may assist the physician in making a diagnosis of a macular hole. The Watzke-Allen test is performed by placing a thin slit-lamp beam directly on the retinal hole during contact-lens biomicroscopic examination. The patient is asked about whether the thin vertical beam of light is interrupted at any point or whether it simply narrows (Figure 9-3). An interruption in the light beam perceived by the patient is a positive Watzke-Allen sign and is useful in diagnosing the presence of a macular hole. A normal-appearing or only narrowed beam is a negative result. The Watzke-Allen sign, however, is of variable consistency particularly in stage 2 macular holes with small retinal dehiscences.

The laser aiming beam spot is also a useful test for assessing the presence or absence of a full-thickness macular hole.[9] The patient is seated at the laser apparatus with a fundus contact lens in place. The 50-µ aiming beam is used to test central areas of the retina focally for visual sensitivity. The inability of the patient to perceive the spot in the area of presumed macular hole is strong evidence for the lack of retinal tissue in that location. In concert with a positive Watzke-Allen sign, this is strong evidence for the presence of a full thickness macular hole.

Ocular coherence tomography (OCT) is a new diagnostic imaging technique for high-resolution imaging of the human retina.[10] Cross-sectional images of optical reflectivity can be obtained with 10-µ longitudinal resolution. This degree of resolution is superior to that of other currently available diagnostic instruments. The high-resolution, cross-sectional images can provide useful clinical information in the differential diagnosis and staging of macular holes.

Surgical Technique

Vitrectomy

MHS usually is performed under local anesthetic on an outpatient basis. Instruments necessary for MHS are listed in Table 9-4. The vitreous surgery is done using standard 20-gauge three-port incisions with infusion cannula, endoillumination, and vitrectomy probe. The vitrectomy proceeds from anterior to posterior. After surgical removal of the anterior and mid vitreous, it is necessary to identify and remove the attached posterior cortical vitreous.

Separation of the posterior hyaloid from the retinal surface is difficult because of the three characteristics of posterior cortical vitreous: its softness, transparency, and tight adherence to the retina. Because of its softness, the cortical vitreous cannot always be removed in a single sheet. It may fragment into multiple pieces, therefore requiring a more tedious effort from the surgeon. Because of its transparency, the cortical vitreous is close to invisible when it is attached to the retina. Lastly, because of its tight adherence to the retina, high suction forces have to be used.

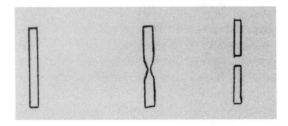

Figure 9-3. Diagram that was given to the patient to determine results of Watzke-Allen sign testing. Choices for response were break (*right*), thinning (*middle*), and no break (*left*). (Reprinted with permission from Martinez J, Smiddy WE, Kim J, Gass JDM. Differentiating macular holes from macular pseudoholes. *Am J Ophthalmol* 1994;117:762–767.)

Table 9-4. Instruments Used for Macular Hole Surgery

- 33-gauge tapered needle
- Soft silicone tip needle (Grieshaber)
- Illuminated pick (Grieshaber)
- Tano membrane stripper (Synergetics)
- Asymmetric forceps (Synergetics)
- Michels pick
- Rice ILM elevator (Synergetics)
- ILM forceps (Grieshaber)
- Membrane forceps/Eckardt (DORC)
- Morris viscoelastic injector

To detect and engage the transparent and tightly adhered posterior cortical vitreous, a soft-tipped silicone extrusion needle can be used. Using active aspiration (150–250 mm Hg) with elevated infusion bottle, the silicone-tipped suction cannula is gently swept over the retinal surface near the major arcades, around the optic nerve or temporal to the macula. The area immediately around the macular hole is avoided because the cuff of the hole is mobile and can be easily incarcerated into the port. When the soft silicone tip engages the cortical vitreous, it is noted to flex. This has been termed the "fish-strike sign" or "divining rod sign" (Figure 9-4). The flexion is typically apparent before the vitreous fibers can be seen. This suction maneuver is safe as long as the vitreous cortex is still present, because the vitreous plugs the port and prevents retinal incarceration and subsequent tearing. However, if the cortex has been unknowingly detached intraoperatively or preoperatively (stage 4 hole), the retina can be aspirated into the port and torn. Once the posterior cortical vitreous is engaged, a posterior vitreous detachment (PVD) can be created with continued suction with anterior-posterior and tangential traction, while moving the tip over the retinal surface. This can also be facilitated by the combined bimanual use of a lighted pick and the soft silicone tip aspiration needle to gently elevate the posterior hyaloid from the retinal surface in a very controlled fashion.

A faster and easier method to remove the posterior vitreous hyaloid is to use the vitreous cutter set on "suction only," directing the port posteriorly and gently sweeping over and around the optic nerve until cortical vitreous fibers are visualized streaming into the port. The cutter's larger port engages the vitreous more firmly and is more efficient at peeling the cortex from the optic nerve. Once this has been accomplished, the vitreous will usually separate easily to the posterior vitreous base. Caution should be exercised once the vitreous has separated from the posterior pole, as retinal tears may develop with excessive traction.

Once the posterior hyaloidal dissection has been initiated, the vitreous cortex becomes visible as a thickened translucent sheet, especially with oblique illumination. Occasionally, the nasal or disc attachments are so firm that the vitreous cutter (on suction only), tissue forceps, or pick manipulation is required to complete the PVD in these areas. It is common to create small disc and retinal hemorrhages during this process. Frequently, a pseudo-operculum can be detected as a luteal-colored fragment attached to the vitreous cortex. A ring of condensed vitreous (Weiss' ring) is observed over the disc corresponding to previous vitreopapillary attachments. Vitreous cutting should be limited until a complete PVD is present to avoid leaving islands of attached posterior cortical vitreous. Once

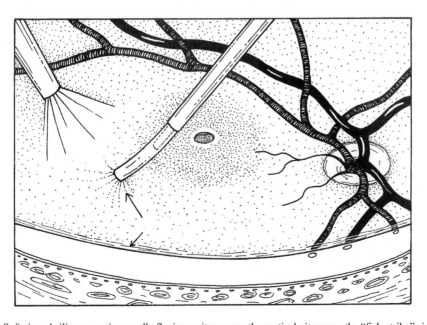

Figure 9-4. Soft-tipped silicone suction needle flexing as it engages the cortical vitreous—the "fish-strike" sign.

the vitreous is completely detached, the vitreous cutter is used to complete the vitrectomy. If residual attached vitreous cortex is present in the posterior pole, it becomes apparent during completion of the air-fluid exchange as a gelatinous substance on the retinal surface.

ERM Removal

Histopathologic studies have shown that the majority of macular holes studied postmortem have associated epiretinal membranes (ERMs). Although ERMs typically appear with later-stage holes and holes of longer duration, they are also common in stage 2 holes.

These ERMs are unlike typical ERMs from other causes. They tend to be finer and more friable and at times are densely adhered to the retina. It may be difficult to distinguish an ERM from internal limiting membrane (ILM) contraction. Often we use a bent microvitreoretinal (MVR) blade or Tano membrane scratcher to create an edge in the ERM, allowing the introduction of a membrane pick. The free edge is grasped with diamond-dusted intraocular tissue forceps and stripped. The ERMs may surround the hole for 360 degrees or can involve only a few clock hours. If present for 360 degrees, they are often tightly adhered to the edge of the hole. At times, this attachment requires cutting to avoid tearing the edge of the hole.

During this maneuver, it is common to create numerous small hemorrhages around the hole. Caution is needed to avoid damaging the inner retina; an early sign of which may be the development of fluffy whitish areas. To avoid phototoxic injury, care is taken to avoid prolonged intense illumination from the light pipe held near the macula.

Internal Limiting Membrane Removal

In the absence of a significant amount of ERM that could be removed, some investigators advocate the removal of the ILM to increase the success rate in closing macular holes.[11] This modification in surgical technique to intentional removal of ILM has been controversial. The advocates of this technique hypothesize that the greater success in closing macular holes with this modified technique is because the removal of the ILM mobilizes the retina around the macular hole so that it is more flexible or elastic. In one nonrandomized, controlled study,[11] 98% of the macular holes were successfully closed with this technique, while only 70% among the control eyes were closed. Additionally, there appeared to be no damaging effect on the vision from the intentional removal of the ILM.

The first step of ILM removal is puncturing ILM with a sharp-tipped MVR blade in the superior macula (Figure 9-5A), about 1 disc diameter away from the macular hole in an 11 o'clock position in both right and left eyes. Once the ILM is punctured the MVR blade is withdrawn from the opening. To assist in visualization of the ILM, Tornambe has suggested using intravitreal Indocyanine Green (ICG) dye, which binds to the ILM and facilitates its visualization intraoperatively (personal communication).

The Rice ILM elevator or Michel's pick is introduced, with the tip directed tangentially into the opening in the ILM and beneath it (Figure 9-5B). The elevator is advanced slightly in an effort to engage only the ILM and not the nerve fiber layer (NFL). Positioning the ILM elevator in the proper plane often is very difficult and sometimes takes several minutes of advancing the tip slightly and withdrawing it if it is not beneath the ILM or if it passes into the NFL. Once the proper dissection plane is established, the ILM elevator is advanced in a clockwise or counter clockwise direction (Figures 9-5C,D). Every effort is made to tunnel beneath the ILM, creating a pocket, and not to create a broad-based sheet of dissected ILM. An intermittent slight lifting motion is used to lift the ILM off the NFL ahead of the instrument tip, to avoid burrowing the tip into the NFL. The ILM is often not visible over the instrument tip, but a slight movement of the retina in the direction of the ILM elevator indicates that it has been engaged. The Morris viscoelastic injector can also be used to facilitate ILM removal by using a viscoelastic to dissect the ILM from the retinal surface mechanically (personal communication). Once the ILM is elevated off at least from one side of the macula, it can be grasped with ILM forceps and peeled off the rest of the central macula, including the margins of the macular hole (Figure 9-5E). The ILM is then grasped more centrally and gently separated from attachments to the margins of the hole.

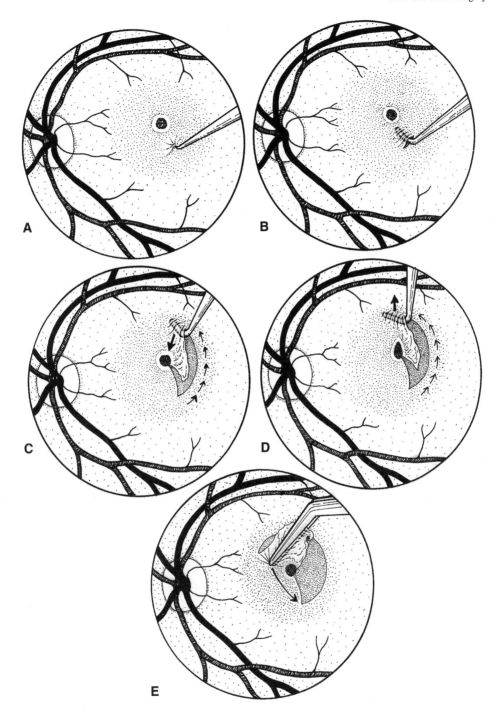

Figure 9-5. A–E, Internal limiting membrane removal.

Air-Fluid Exchange

After careful examination of the peripheral retina for retinal tears with an indirect ophthalmoscope, a total air-fluid exchange is performed. Because dehydration of the retinal surface may be associated with visual field defects following macular hole surgery, we no longer wait to exhaustively remove all of the intraocular fluid.

Once all fluid has been removed over the disc, the residual fluid in the base of the macular hole is aspirated using a 33-gauge metal tapered-tip aspiration needle. Care is taken to avoid "bumping" the RPE. The edges of the macular hole will tend to remain on the pigment epithelium as this is completed. Frequently, the edges appear to slide closer together at this stage; this is considered a good prognostic sign. In apparent eccentric stage 2 eyes, no attempt is made to drain the fluid in the base of the hole, for fear of causing progression of the hole to stage 3.

Tamponade

Long-Acting Gas

A nonexpansile concentration of long-acting gas is exchanged for the air. We have most frequently used 20% sulfur hexafluoride (SF_6), although longer-acting gases such as perfluoropropane (C_3F_8) have been used in cases in which compliance with prone positioning is difficult. Thompson et al.[12] have reported anatomic success in 53% of patients in which air alone was used versus 97% in which 16% C_3F_8 was used. The visual success rates were 20% and 62%, respectively. A subsequent study[13] showed that the success rate with 5% and 10% of C_3F_8 (shorter-acting bubble) was only 65% as compared to 94% with 16% C_3F_8. Recently, Park et al.[14] have reported good surgical results with the use of intravitreous air, along with a shorter 4-day duration of strict *face-down* positioning. Tornambe has also reported good surgical results using long-acting gas without face-down positioning. It is important, however, to realize that face-down positioning theoretically increases the buoyancy effect of gas bubbles that may augment the surface tension effects of intraocular gas tamponades that in turn may enhance anatomic closure of macular holes in most patients.

In those unusual situations in which general anesthesia is used, it is critical that administration of nitrous oxide be stopped at least 15–30 minutes before air-gas exchange.

Silicone Oil

In patients who are either unable or unwilling to comply with the strict 1-week face-down positioning postoperatively, liquid silicone can be used instead of long-acting gas as an extended intraocular tamponade. However, silicone oil tamponade has two disadvantages: (1) an increased potential for cataract formation, and (2) it requires a second surgery to remove the oil.

After the fluid-air exchange is performed, an air-silicone oil exchange is performed by injecting silicone into the air-filled eye (with the air pump on) until silicone oil reaches the level of the sclerotomies or the posterior surface of the lens or intraocular lens. Then, the infusion cannula is removed and the sclerotomies are closed. The final intraocular pressure is left between 10 and 15 mm Hg.

The patients are asked to maintain a face-down position as much as possible until the morning of the first postoperative day, following which they are instructed only to avoid extended supine positioning. They may return to normal light activity on the first postoperative day, but are cautioned to avoid strenuous physical exercise.

The silicone oil can be removed 4–8 weeks postoperatively. Oil removal is accomplished either by passive efflux through a cannula or by active aspiration through a 19-gauge, $^3/_8$-inch needle. The eye is meticulously examined for small droplets of residual silicone that are removed through a 19-gauge, thin-walled needle.

Adjuvants

Histopathologic studies have demonstrated that with macular hole resolution after MHS, the edges are reapproximated, and the residual defect filled with fibroglial cells.[15] Furthermore, the pseudo-operculum has been demonstrated in some cases to consist of fibroglial elements rather than photoreceptor elements.[16] The rationale for using adjunctive therapy regimens is the stimulation of fibroglial proliferation to close the hole reproducibly, avoiding trauma to adjacent functional retinal elements.[6] Therefore, adjunctive therapeutic interventions, including biological tissue adhesive, transforming growth factor–beta$_2$ (TGF-β_2), autologous serum, and autologous platelet concentrate, have been investigated to improve success rates in macular hole surgery. The adjuvant is added after a fluid-air exchange has been performed and is placed onto the macular hole via a 33-gauge cannula.

There are controversies in the use of adjunctive therapy. Success rates for macular hole surgery have been improving as a result of greater familiarity with surgical techniques and better case selection. Anatomic success rates in excess of 90%, with parallel visual success rates, among series without adjunctive agents call into question the beneficial role offered by the use of adjunctive therapies. However, the excellent surgical results in most series with adjuvants have been achieved without ILM removal, whereas similar surgical success among those without adjuvants has needed ILM removal. Therefore, the relative ease of the surgical procedures for adjunctive interventions merits consideration of their use.

Biological Tissue Adhesive

The first adjunctive therapy reported was a biological tissue adhesive, a commercially available product composed of bovine thrombin and pooled human fibrinogen. Since then, other investigators have used the strategy of thrombin with a fibrinogen -containing substance, such as autologous plasma, or cryoprecipitate derived from autologous serum. Both series reported anatomic success rates of 80% with higher rates of visual improvement. However, because these and subsequent pilot studies were not randomized and did not have controls, the efficacy of biological tissue adhesives is difficult to judge.

Transforming Growth Factor–Beta

Some investigators have reported improved success rates in macular hole surgery using bovine TGF-β_2. However, the results of a phase III, prospective, randomized, placebo-controlled trial did not show a statistically significant difference between recombinant TGF-β_2 and placebo.[16] Consequently, further investigations have been suspended.

Autologous Serum

Autologous serum has also been investigated. While several investigators have reported anatomic success rates ranging from 80% to 90% in uncontrolled clinical trials, nonrandomized but controlled pilot studies have not shown a treatment benefit.[17]

Autologous Platelet Concentrate

A pilot study using autologous platelet concentrate reported a 95% anatomic success rate. Subsequently, a nonrandomized study demonstrated that the group that underwent autologous platelet concentrate therapy has a significantly higher anatomic success rate than the control group, 95% to 65%.[18] Further well-controlled and randomized studies will be required to determine the efficacy of this as an adjunct.

Combined Cataract Extraction and Intraocular Lens Implantation with Macular Hole Surgery

Many patients develop cataracts after MHS, eventually requiring cataract surgery. Therefore, investigators have looked into the feasibility of combining MHS and cataract surgery by performing them sequentially in the same operative session. One initial report shows that these two procedures can be performed during the same operative session with successful anatomic results and improvement in visual acuity.[19] The advantages of combining the two procedures are patient convenience, decreased surgical expense, and shortened time for visual rehabilitation.

Postoperative Care

Postoperatively, 24-hour-a-day strict prone positioning for 1 week is prescribed (Figure 9-6). This is a significant trial for both patient and family members, and careful patient selection and preoperative counseling is mandatory to ensure cooperation. Families should be given the opportunity to plan ahead to secure such simple items as drinking straws for the patient and for specialized equipment such as massage tables for comfortable prone sleeping (Figure 9-7). Other aids that our patients have found useful include small portable television sets, prism glasses that aid in their head-down ambulation and viewing, analgesics, and anti-inflammatory drugs for back or neck pain. At times, surgery is not recommended because the preoperative evaluation concludes that prone positioning will be too physically taxing for the patient. A possible alternative approach in such cases is use of silicone oil, or long-acting gas without prone positioning.

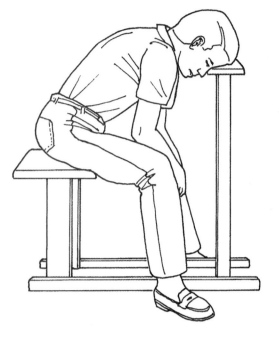

Figure 9-6. Face-down position.

At the 1-week visit, approximately 50% of the gas bubble remains after use of 20% SF_6. If the patient has been truly compliant, it is common to see cellular debris precipitated on the corneal endothelium. We call this a good positioning spot (GPS) (Figure 9-8). This finding may be the only objective measure of actual patient compliance with prone positioning. In the case of primary surgical failure, the absence of a GPS may suggest poor compliance as an etiology. The macula can usually be seen at this visit, and predictions regarding anatomic success can usually be made. If the edges of the macular hole are flattened, anatomic success is the rule. On the other hand, if the edges are still visible and the cuff elevated, anatomic failure occurs despite additional prone positioning.

Complications

Macular hole surgery is accompanied by the same potential complications seen in other vitreoretinal surgical cases. These complications may be considered as perioperative (intraoperative and early postoperative) complications or late postoperative complications (Table 9-5).

Iatrogenic retinal breaks are a relatively common complication of macular hole surgery, occurring in 2–17% of cases.[20] They most likely develop during the mechanical stripping of the cortical vitreous. Gentle manipulation of the vitreous at this step will reduce this complication. The majority of the breaks are peripheral. Thus, it is important to carefully examine for retinal breaks prior to fluid-air exchange (using indirect ophthalmoscopy with scleral depression), as small breaks are easily overlooked when the vitreous cavity is filled with air. The retinal tears are treated with cryotherapy or laser and fluid-air exchange, with appropriate postoperative positioning.

Rhegmatogenous retinal detachments have a reported frequency of less than 3% in most large series. In some instances, they have been noted in up to 14–25% of the cases. Again, thorough examination of the retina prior to the fluid-air exchange will identify the retinal detachments and ensure that all detachments are appropriately treated.

A third perioperative complication is increased intraocular pressure. Increased intraocular pressure after macular hole surgery has been reported in up to one-third of eyes.[8] This effect does not relate to the type or concentration of gas used, or the duration of gas tamponade, but was found to be dramatically higher in patients who received recombinant TGF-β_2. Angle-closure glaucoma has been reported in two studies and was treated successfully with laser iridotomy in both instances.

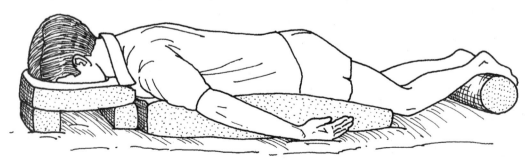

Figure 9-7. Prone sleeping position.

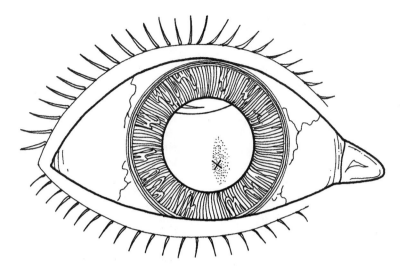

Figure 9-8. The "good positioning spot" seen on the corneal endothelium indicates appropriate postoperative patient positioning.

Table 9-5. Complications of Macular Hole Surgery

Perioperative
   a. Iatrogenic retinal breaks
   b. Rhegmatogenous retinal detachments
   c. Increased intraocular pressure
   d. Endophthalmitis

Late Postoperative
   a. Reopening of the macular hole
   b. Visual field defects
   c. Progressive nuclear sclerosis
   d. Macular pigmentary changes
   e. Cystoid macular edema
   f. Vascular occlusion: AION, BRAO, CRAO
   g. Choroidal neovascular membrane

Late postoperative complications include reopening of the macular hole, visual field defects, progressive nuclear sclerosis, and retinal pigmentary changes. Macular holes reopen in approximately 2–4% of cases.[21,22] Visual field defects occur most commonly in the inferior temporal location. The etiology of this complication is poorly understood. It has been speculated that the visual field loss may be due to nerve fiber layer damage that occurs during extended fluid-gas exchange and subsequent retinal dehydration,[6] or possibly damage to the peripapillary nerve fiber bundle during the separation of the posterior vitreous from the retinal surface. Progression of nuclear sclerotic cataracts is the most common complication of macular hole surgery, as in series of vitrectomies for conditions other than macular holes. Studies have reported incidence of nuclear sclerotic cataract progression in the range of 13–95% after MHS.[20] Although the precise etiology of the progressive nuclear sclerosis is unknown, altered lens metabolism after vitrectomy is believed to play a role.[20] Poor positioning also increases contact between the gas bubble and the lens capsule, which facilitates cataract formation. Other risk factors are increased patient age and increased time interval after surgery. This complication is managed by cataract surgery and lens implantation. Finally, retinal pigment epithelial changes have been described and have been attributed to phototoxicity, mechanical damage to the pigment epithelium during suction of subretinal fluid through the macular hole, and pressure effects of the gas bubble on the choriocapillaris and pigment epithelium during prolonged face-down positioning.[23] Later series in which prolonged illumination of the foveal area with the fiberoptic illuminator was avoided have noted this finding less frequently.[6] Other rare complications included cystoid macular edema, vascular occlusion, choroidal neovascular membrane, postoperative endophthalmitis, and ulnar nerve paralysis.

Conclusion

Vitrectomy is an effective procedure for closure of macular hole. While a variety of modifications in surgical technique have been reported, the same basic principles are present in all methods used. The main objective is to remove anterior-posterior and tangential tractions, which cause a central retinal dehiscence that eventually leads to formation of a macular hole. A complete pars plana vitrectomy is performed with elevation and removal of the posterior cortical vitreous. Any epiretinal membrane should be removed. Some surgeons also advocate the removal of the internal limiting membrane (ILM). The retinal periphery is carefully examined by indirect ophthalmoscopy, and a fluid-air exchange is performed, followed by exchange of the air with a long-acting gas. In selected patients who are not good candidates for surgery with gas, the use of silicone oil provides an alternative for surgical repair.

Some investigators have reported a greater than 90% success rate in macular hole closure by more aggressively peeling off the ILM at the time of macular hole surgery. Others have reported achieving similar results by using a variety of adjuvants, including autologous serum, autologous plasma or cryoprecipitate with bovine thrombin, and autologous platelet concentrate without ILM removal to improve closure rates of primary idiopathic macular holes, as well as to close reopened holes.

Regardless of the technique used to repair the macular hole, it is widely recognized that strict postoperative face-down positioning is a successful technique used by most surgeons. Face-down positioning helps to effectively tamponade the macular hole and promotes macular hole closure. The continual improvement of techniques and early surgical intervention has indeed made this a gratifying procedure.

References*

1. **Kelly NE, Wendel RT. Vitreous surgery for idiopathic macular hole. *Arch Ophthalmol* 1991;109: 654–659.**
2. Yuzawa M, Watanabe A, Takahashi Y, Matsui M. Observation of idiopathic full-thickness macular holes. Follow-up observation. *Arch Ophthalmol* 1994;112: 1051–1056.
3. de Bustros S. Impending macular holes. In: Madreperla SA, McCuen II BW, eds. *Macular Hole: Pathogenesis, Diagnosis, and Treatment.* Boston: Butterworth-Heinemann; 1999:89–94.
4. Rubin JS, Glaser BM, Thompson JT, et al. Vitrectomy, fluid-gas exchange and transforming growth factor beta-2 for the treatment of macular holes. *Ophthalmology* 1995;102:1840–1845.
5. **Huang SS, Wendel RT. Vitreous surgery for full-thickness macular holes. In: Madreperla SA, McCuen II BW, eds. *Macular Hole: Pathogenesis, Diagnosis, and Treatment.* Boston: Butterworth-Heinemann; 1999:95–104.**
6. **Smiddy WE. Pharmacologic adjuncts and macular hole surgery. In: Madreperla SA, McCuen II BW, eds. *Macular Hole: Pathogenesis, Diagnosis, and Treatment.* Boston: Butterworth-Heinemann; 1999: 105–114.**
7. Ryan EH, Gilbert HD. Results of surgical treatment of recent-onset full-thickness idiopathic macular holes. *Arch Ophthalmol* 1994;112:545–553.
8. Haller JA. Clinical characteristics and epidemiology of macular holes. In: Madreperla SA, McCuen II BW, eds. *Macular Hole: Pathogenesis, Diagnosis, and Treatment.* Boston: Butterworth-Heinemann; 1999:25–36.
9. Martinez J, Smiddy WE, Kim J, Gass JDM. Differentiating macular holes from macular pseudoholes. *Am J Ophthalmol* 1994;117:762–767.
10. Hee MR, Puliafito CA, Wong C, et al. Optical coherence tomography of macular holes. *Ophthalmology* 1995;102:748–756.
11. Rice TA. Internal limiting membrane removal in surgery for full-thickness macular holes. In: Madreperla SA, McCuen II BW, eds. *Macular Hole: Pathogenesis, Diagnosis, and Treatment.* Boston: Butterworth-Heinemann; 1999:125–146.
12. Thompson JT, Glaser BM, Sjaarda RN, et al. Effects of intraocular bubble duration in the treatment of macular holes by vitrectomy and transforming growth factor–β_2. *Ophthalmology* 1994;101:1195–1200.
13. Thompson JT, Smiddy WE, Glaser BM, et al. Intraocular tamponade duration and success of macular hole surgery. *Retina* 1996;16:373–382.
14. Park DW, Sipperley JO, Sneed SR, et al. Macular hole surgery with internal-limiting membrane peeling and intravitreous air. *Ophthalmology* 1999;106(7):1392–1397.
15. Funata M, Wendel RT, de la Cruz Z, Green WR. Clinicopathologic study of bilateral macular holes treated with pars plana vitrectomy and gas tamponade. *Retina* 1992;12:289–298.
16. Thompson JT, Smiddy WE, Williams GA, et al. Comparison of recombinant TGF-β_2 and placebo as an adjunctive agent for macular hole surgery. *Ophthalmology* 1998;105:700–706.
17. Ezra E, Wells JA, Charteris DG, et al. Macular hole surgery with and without autologous serum: a prospective study of 109 consecutive eyes. *Invest Ophthalmol Vis Sci* 1996;37:S474.

---

*Bold references indicate suggested reading as well.

18. Gaudric A, Massin P, Paques M, et al. Autologous platelet concentrate for the treatment of full-thickness macular holes. *Graefes Arch Clin Exp Ophthalmol* 1995;233:549–554.

19. Miller JH, Googe JM, Hoskins JC. Combined macular hole and cataract surgery. *Am J Ophthalmol* 1997; 123(5):705–707.

20. Pendergast SD, Williams GA. Complications of macular hole surgery. In: Madreperla SA, McCuen II BW, eds. *Macular Hole: Pathogenesis, Diagnosis, and Treatment.* Boston: Butterworth-Heinemann; 1999:155–168.

21. **Freeman WR, Azen SP, Kim JW, et al. Vitrectomy for the treatment of full-thickness stage 3 or 4 macular holes. Results of a multicentered randomized clinical trial. The vitrectomy for treatment of macular hole study group. *Arch Ophthalmol* 1997; 115:11–21.**

22. **Duker JS, Wendel RT, Patel AC, Puliafito CA. Late reopening of macular holes following initial successful vitreous surgery. *Ophthalmology* 1994;101: 1373–1378.**

23. **Kokame GT. Vitrectomy for macular hole: the randomized multicenter clinical trials. In: Madreperla SA, McCuen II BW, eds. *Macular Hole: Pathogenesis, Diagnosis, and Treatment.* Boston: Butterworth-Heinemann; 1999:115–124.**

10

Complications and Postoperative Management

Mark S. Blumenkranz

The primary objective of retinal reattachment surgery is to restore normal anatomic relationships between the neurosensory retina and the retinal pigment epithelium (RPE) by methods that result in the maintenance or maximal restoration of central and peripheral visual function. Experienced retinal surgeons using the techniques outlined in previous chapters of this book can achieve this objective in the majority of cases with a single operation and a minimum number of complications. Complications are undesirable for two reasons: (1) they may lessen the chances for retinal reattachment with a single operation (as in the case of retinal incarceration) or (2) they may result in reduced visual function in cases in which anatomic retinal reattachment is achieved (as in the case of subretinal hemorrhage). As in all surgical disciplines, the most effective treatment for surgical complications is to avoid them. By using atraumatic surgical technique and following established surgical principles, complications can be minimized.

Complications of retinal reattachment surgery can be broadly grouped into those that occur in the *intraoperative environment* or those in the *postoperative period*. The latter can in turn be classified into *early* and *late* complications, with the former being the major subject of this chapter.

Intraoperative Complications

Penetration with Scleral Suture

The necessity of achieving adequate length and depth of scleral bites to produce suitable buckle height has already been addressed in Chapter 7. Occasionally, especially in myopic eyes or those with localized radial staphylomata, the needle will penetrate the choroid and pigment epithelium. This risk can be reduced by using a spatula rather than a cutting needle. In eyes in which the retina is sufficiently detached in that quadrant, subretinal fluid will be released as the needle hub is withdrawn from the scleral pass, with immediate softening of the globe. If the retina is attached in that quadrant, no outward sign may occur although occasionally a small bead of vitreous may be seen at the site. In either case, if blood emanates from the needle tract externally, the suture must be immediately but carefully removed from the tract after cutting it close to the sclera to reduce the chance of intravitreal or subretinal bleeding. The site should then be carefully inspected by indirect ophthalmoscopy and treated by cryopexy or indirect laser if there is evidence of a traumatic retinal tear. If there is evidence of localized subretinal hemorrhage, the intraocular pressure should be increased and the eye and head positioned so that extension of hemorrhage into the macula is either avoided or minimized. If there is no evidence of external or internal bleeding from the perforation site, it is advisable to proceed with placement of the additional scleral sutures. Care should be taken to avoid another accidental perforation in the soft, already predisposed eye. When all the additional sutures have been placed, and the globe temporarily buckled to restore a more normal intraocular pressure, it may be advisable to replace the defective suture 1–2 mm beyond the first bite (either anteriorly or posteriorly) such that the original perforation site is now encompassed in the buckle. In some cases, subretinal fluid drainage may no longer be necessary, although as a general rule it is unwise to evacuate subretinal fluid forcibly from an inadvertent drain site, because of the risk of hemorrhage.

Rupture of the Globe Wall

Occasionally in eyes that have undergone prior retinal procedures, trauma, or high myopia, a gaping defect may occur intraoperatively that results in massive loss of vitreous and deflation. Areas of thin sclera (such as beneath the insertions of the recti muscles) are particularly prone to this complication. In such instances the most expeditious course is to oversew the defect with a 6-0 or 7-0 absorbable or an 8-0 nylon suture if the hole is not too large. For larger defects the entire area can be covered with an appropriately trimmed explant held in place by horizontal mattress sutures secured in more normal surrounding sclera. The globe is then reinflated with balanced salt solution or air and the remainder of the operation resumed. In rare instances, the use of cyanoacrylate glue, processed pericardium, or bank sclera may be considered.

Inability to Drain Subretinal Fluid Successfully

In some cases the surgeon may not be able to evacuate subretinal fluid successfully or safely because of its shallowness in an accessible scleral site, engorgement or detachment of the choroid, nearby chorioretinal scars, or other factors. In such instances it is highly recommended that the surgeon revise the operative plan and consider other tech-

niques, including conventional nondrainage and the placement of an intravitreal gas bubble, since drainage complications including incarceration, retinal hole formation, and subretinal hemorrhage tend to be the most frequent and severe intraoperative complications.

Retinal Incarceration in the Drain Site

During the course of release of subretinal fluid through a drainage sclerotomy, the retina may become incarcerated in the choroidal puncture site and occasionally prolapse externally or blow out if the complication is not promptly recognized. The likelihood of this is increased by the following factors: selection of a drainage site beneath shallowly detached retina, excessive pressure on the globe during drainage, or creation of too large a defect in the choroid. It should be immediately suspected when the surgeon notes an abrupt cessation of previously brisk fluid drainage, often immediately preceded by a small burst of external pigment. It can be confirmed ophthalmoscopically when the retina shows starfolds and is engaged in the underlying drain site.

Prior to the ophthalmoscopic examination, some surgeons prefer that the drainage site be closed by temporarily tying either the overlying buckle suture (so that the explant covers the drainage site) or the preplaced sclerotomy mattress suture (if one was used; see Chapter 7).

Once an incarceration has been identified, the surgeon may attempt to reverse this by reducing pressure on the globe and simultaneously averting and pulling the lips of the sclerotomy outward. In some cases in which the retina is not frankly prolapsed externally, gentle external pressure with a blunt muscle hook or a stream of balanced salt solution may be successful. In most cases these maneuvers are unsuccessful and the surgeon must determine whether a retinal hole has also been created that requires an adhesive modality such as cryopexy or indirect laser. In most cases of irreversible incarceration, the site is already in the bed of a planned buckle, so no further modification is required. If not, however, scleral buckling of this site is strongly advised. I routinely apply cryopexy to all accidental incarceration sites since, in many instances, it may facilitate the identification of small retinal defects. Larger retinal defects in incarceration sites are readily recognized by the appearance of translucent vascularized retinal tissue or a burst of liquid vitreous from the site. In some instances, a late incarceration may be created after otherwise successful drainage of subretinal fluid during buckle manipulation if the drain site has not been previously closed. For this reason as well as potential reoperation, I choose to close all drain sites with a preplaced absorbable suture such as 7-0 Vicryl. The major complications of retinal incarceration (aside from retinal breaks) are the creation of radial retinal folds that interfere with buckling of other tears in the early postoperative period and localized or generalized retinal proliferation (macular pucker, starfolds, and proliferative vitreoretinopathy [PVR]) in the later postoperative period.

Subretinal Hemorrhage

Another complication that may occur during drainage of subretinal fluid is intraocular hemorrhage, usually into the subretinal space. Factors that favor the development of this complication include highly myopic eyes, actively inflamed eyes, posteriorly selected (and midquadrant) drain sites, and the use of overly large, sharp drainage instruments. The likelihood of developing this complication can be reduced by selecting a drainage site as anterior as possible beneath adequately detached retina in the 3, 6, 9, and 12 o'clock meridians, which has the effect of avoiding the drainage beds of the vortex veins and their immediate larger tributaries. Once the sclerotomy has been performed, the underlying choroidal knuckle is carefully inspected (preferably with magnification) to ensure that there are no large choroidal vessels in the region. If any doubt exists, transillumination may be used. I, generally, lightly diathermize the choroidal bed to reduce further the risk of accidental hemorrhage, although this is probably not necessary if the bed has been carefully inspected and found to be free of large vessels. The development of a subretinal hemorrhage from a drainage site is usually, but not always, heralded by external bleeding. External bleeding from the drain site mandates that the surgeon promptly inspect the drain site internally by indirect ophthalmoscopy before proceeding further with drainage. If blood is seen internally at the drain site or posteriorly, light diathermy should be applied externally to the drain site, the drain site

closed, the intraocular pressure normalized by external pressure on the globe with a cotton-tipped applicator, and a new drain site selected. If blood has tracked beneath the detached macula, some consideration should be given to appropriate positioning of the globe or head so that the blood may migrate gravitationally to an inferior extramacular location. This positioning should be continued in the immediate postoperative period. In the case of a large submacular hemorrhage in an eye with total or inferior subtotal detachment, it may be justified to defer further drainage and use a pneumatic technique in conjunction with reverse Trendelenburg positioning to facilitate movement of blood to a more inferior extramacular location overnight. In rare instances of bullous hemorrhagic macular detachment occurring as a complication of scleral buckling, vitrectomy and fluid-air exchange with or without internal drainage of the hemorrhage may reduce late blood-related macular dysfunction, although this technique remains unproven and controversial. In general the natural history of submacular hemorrhage following choroidal perforation during scleral buckling is more benign than other clinical syndromes such as age-related macular degeneration.

Acute Ocular Hypertension

Acute rises in the intraocular pressure (IOP) are frequently encountered in the course of retinal reattachment surgery. Most frequently the IOP elevation is the result of a buckle-induced compression of the globe or injection of a vitreous bubble to promote break tamponade. Under normal physiologic circumstances, the outflow facility of the eye is able to compensate for these acute pressure rises, with the rate of aqueous outflow proportional to the IOP and thereby increased. In the case of expansile concentrations of insoluble gases such as sulfur hexafluoride and perfluoropropane, the concomitant use of nitrous oxide (which is also highly insoluble) as a general anesthetic agent may lead to severe and unpredictable IOP increases related to the equilibrium-driven accumulation of nitrous oxide within the intraocular gas bubble. This complication can be avoided by advising the anesthesiologist when expansile gases may be used and avoiding the use of nitrous oxide in such cases. When nitrous oxide has been used, it is highly recommended that the anesthesiologist switch to another inhalational agent at least 10–15 minutes prior to the instillation of intravitreal gas. Experimental studies on rabbits indicate that when outflow facility is normal, elevation of the IOP acutely to levels of 100 mm Hg by intravitreal injection of a 0.4-cc gas bubble is followed by normalization of the IOP in 60 minutes or less. It is also known that placement of an encircling buckle reduces the outflow facility of the eye, at least temporarily, and thus may exacerbate the tendency toward ocular hypertension both intraoperatively and postoperatively. This can be offset by several methods including preoperative intermittent compression of the globe to lower the IOP, preoperative or intraoperative treatment with a carbonic anhydrase inhibitor (such as acetazolamide 500 mg) or a hyperosmotic agent (such as intravenous mannitol 1g/kg) and, most commonly, paracentesis. A general rule of thumb is that the normal eye will tolerate an IOP that does not result in closure of the central retinal artery for more than 50% of the duration of the cardiac cycle. This guideline should not be applied to eyes with preexisting glaucoma or ischemic ocular disease.

One special technique I have found helpful in rare situations in which the ability to perform encirclage and intravitreal gas injection is effectively precluded by IOP considerations is to remove a small amount of vitreous. This is performed under indirect ophthalmoscopic control with a mechanized cutter positioned in the midvitreous cavity without the need for a separate infusion port or light pipe. Sufficient volume is created to permit safe encirclage and gas injection, although potential complications include the creation of radial retinal folds, and accidental lens or retinal damage unless the surgeon is experienced with the technique. I find this technique preferable to needle aspiration of vitreous, which is more unreliable and prone to the creation of vitreous tracts (and possibly increased vitreoretinal traction).

Retinal Fold Development

Radial retinal folds develop in eyes undergoing encircling procedures with drainage of subretinal fluid because the equatorial scleral circumference of the globe is shortened proportionally more than the equatorial retinal circumference. The radial fold represents pleating of the retina to accommodate its new scleral circumference and appears to occur pref-

erentially in meridians containing retinal breaks. In addition to their potential involvement of the macula and aesthetic considerations, retinal folds are undesirable because they often contribute to continued movement of subretinal fluid through the retinal break. They can be avoided in many instances by limiting the degree of circumferential scleral shortening induced by shortening (i.e., tightening) the encircling band and injecting a quantity of intravitreal air or gas when a large amount of subretinal fluid has been evacuated. The instillation of intravitreal air has the dual benefit of both restoring the intravitreal volume (and pressure) to a more normal level without excessive band shortening, and providing postoperative tamponade for a retinal break should a retinal fold occur through a break, causing so-called fish-mouthing (see Chapter 7). Another approach to the problem of fish-mouthing is the placement of a radial buckle beneath the radial fold, although this technique is not generally applicable to eyes with multiple retinal folds and is in general less desirable than the use of air or gas.

Early Postoperative Complications (First 72 Hours)

Persistence of Subretinal Fluid

When all subretinal fluid has been drained intraoperatively, it is uncommon for any to be present on the morning after surgery if all the breaks have been identified and appropriately treated. In instances in which not all the subretinal fluid can be successfully or easily drained, or in nondrainage procedures, subretinal fluid may still persist on the first postoperative day. If the breaks appear appropriately positioned overlying the buckle and the amount of fluid is either equal to or less than that observed at the termination of the operation the patient may be safely observed for evidence of further subretinal fluid reabsorption, which generally occurs. If (1) there appears to be more subretinal fluid than present at the termination of the procedure, (2) a prominent retinal fold communicates between the retinal break and subretinal fluid posterior to the buckle, (3) the retinal break is marginally positioned on the buckle, (4) the retinal break is very large (and not well supported), (5) the macula is still detached, (6) there is clinical evidence of continued vitreous traction on the retinal break, or (7) if retinal breaks have not settled in an eye that has been previously vitrectomized, and there is not already a bubble present, I favor an intravitreal injection of air or an expansile gas within the first 48–72 hours. This is most effective if the tear is located within the superior 8 hours of the fundus (or in the posterior pole). The procedure can be performed at the patient's bedside, in a minor surgical suite, or in a reclining examination chair, with minimal additional risk and invariably results in complete subretinal fluid reabsorption unless severe vitreoretinal traction is present. The technique is outlined in the following section.

Exudative Retinal Detachment

Scleral buckling surgery, when combined with heavy cryopexy, can lead to the accumulation of exudative subretinal fluid 48–72 hours following surgery. The subretinal fluid tends to be turbid (obscuring choroidal detail) and shifting in location; it tends to accumulate posterior to the buckle and not contiguous to retinal breaks. Short courses of systemic steroids are effective in treating this complication.

Ocular Hypertension

It is not uncommon to see mild to moderate ocular hypertension (IOP 25–30 mm Hg) with an open angle occurring on the first or second postoperative day, especially in eyes undergoing encircling procedures. These can be successfully treated with a topical β-blocker for the first week or two after surgery, with little risk of optic nerve damage in the otherwise normal eye. Patients with known preexisting glaucoma or a compromised angle should be pretreated with a β-blocker and/or carbonic anhydrase inhibitor to minimize expected fluctuations in the IOP. When the IOP is greater than 35 on the first or second day after surgery the most common cause in phakic patients is the concomitant development of choroidal detachment (see below). In most cases the angle remains open although there may be mild to moderate shallowing. Treatment consists of pupillary dilation, topical steroids, a β-blocker, and topical or oral carbonic anhydrase inhibitor if necessary. Patients may rarely develop true angle closure glau-

coma after scleral buckling. Most often this occurs in pseudophakic patients with anterior chamber lenses, and is accompanied by frank iris bombe and, frequently, pupillary seclusion. The primary treatment is vigorous pupillary dilation to relieve the seclusion. If this is unsuccessful, laser iridectomies with the YAG or argon laser are usually successful in relieving the block, although multiple iridectomies in different secluded quadrants and, occasionally, vitreolysis behind the iridectomy, may be required. If all of these measures are unsuccessful, pars plana vitrectomy and iridectomy will invariably relieve the problem in the absence of large choroidal detachments. Some phakic patients (with either preexisting uveitis or postoperative anterior segment ischemia) or aphakic and pseudophakic patients may develop pupillary seclusion, iris bombe, and acute IOP elevation as the result of a pupillary fibrin membrane (discussed in a subsequent section).

Choroidal Detachment

Along with mild ocular hypertension, serous choroidal detachment is probably the most frequent complication of scleral buckling procedures, occurring in approximately 25% of cases. The likelihood of postoperative choroidal detachment is increased with increasing patient age, the use of an encircling buckle, posterior placement of scleral buckles (compromising vortex veins), and drainage of subretinal fluid. Although the development of serous choroidal detachment is not associated with a decreased long-term retinal reattachment rate, it is frequently associated with moderate to severe elevation of the IOP and may be related to mildly reduced levels of central vision in long-term follow-up studies. Choroidal detachments may be annular and difficult to detect (often associated with mild to moderate shallowing of the anterior chamber) or lobular and variable in size. In general, the treatment for mild to moderate choroidal detachment is conservative, consisting of cycloplegics and topical steroids. In some cases, oral steroids are used if considerable inflammation is present. In rare instances, it may be necessary to drain serous choroidal detachments if they are "kissing" or associated with severe compromise of anterior structures such as a malpositioned lens. Surgical therapy consists of a radial or winged scleral incision overlying the pars plana to the plane of the supra-choroidal space. I have found the simultaneous intraocular infusion of air with an automated pump helpful. In the case of kissing choroidal detachments, some consideration should be given to repositioning the buckle to a more anterior location, if possible, to reduce vortex vein compression.

Fibrinoid Reaction and
Anterior Segment Ischemia

When fibrinoid reaction is present in the anterior chamber on the first postoperative day following a scleral buckling procedure in a nonuveitic eye, it generally signifies that anterior segment ischemia has occurred. This is frequently accompanied by choroidal detachment and ocular hypertension. Patients with preexisting retinal vascular compromise, especially those with sickle cell anemia or the acute retinal necrosis syndrome, are particularly prone to this complication. In the otherwise noncompromised eye the likelihood of anterior segment ischemia or necrosis is increased by the use of an excessively high or broad encircling scleral buckle producing vortex vein compromise. In patients with predisposing retinal vascular disease, the frequency of this serious complication can be reduced by avoiding encirclage if possible, being certain the intraocular tension is not excessively elevated at the termination of surgery, and avoiding vortex vein compromise during orbital dissection and buckle placement.

The other signs of anterior segment ischemia, in addition to fibrinoid reaction, include corneal epithelial and stromal edema out of proportion to the intraocular pressure, keratic precipitates (usually pigmented), iris atrophy and liberation of pigment into the anterior chamber, acute cataract, and occasionally pupillary eccentricity. The treatment of choice is reduction of the IOP and vigorous topical and, in some instances, systemic steroid therapy. In cases where extremely large choroidal detachments are also present, some consideration may be given to replacing the buckling element and draining the choroidal detachments within the first 24–48 hours.

Fibrinoid response in the anterior chamber is not infrequently seen in eyes undergoing both scleral buckling and vitrectomy (see Chapter 8) in the absence of anterior segment ischemia. It most frequently occurs in diabetic patients with extensive ocular neovascularization, trauma patients, and patients with the acute retinal necrosis syndrome, although any patient with intraocular oozing of blood in the immediate postoperative period may manifest this response. In this instance, treatment is not required unless either secondary complications of the fibrin ensue (such as pupillary block) or clear visualization of the posterior segment is required for additional maneuvers such as laser photocoagulation. The intracameral injection of 10–25 micrograms of recombinant tissue plasminogen activator (tPA) is the preferred treatment for this condition, if severe. Mild cases of pupillary fibrin usually resolve spontaneously without serious sequelae.

Cataract

The development of acute cataractous change in the immediate postoperative period following scleral buckling is uncommon and almost invariably related to the use of intraocular gas in the absence of signs of anterior segment ischemia. The mechanism may be either through mechanical damage during intravitreal gas injection or the indirect effects of gas on the lens. In general, in eyes not undergoing vitrectomy with injection of a subtotal gas bubble, these effects are transient and not associated with an unfavorable long-term prognosis. In eyes with larger, long-acting bubbles of perfluoropropane gas, especially after vitrectomy, feathery posterior cortical opacities or vacuolar posterior epithelial changes resembling fish scales may occur. These are also generally transient although they frequently herald the development of a late posterior subcapsular or nuclear sclerotic cataract. Late nuclear sclerosis is a very frequent complication in patients over the age of 40 undergoing vitrectomy alone or in conjunction with scleral buckling, whether or not intraocular gas has been used.

If cataract is not accompanied by acute lens swelling and compromise of anterior segment structures, treatment is not required immediately unless clear visualization of the posterior segment is required for additional postoperative maneuvers. In instances where there is accidental mechanical trauma to the lens, acute swelling of the lens may occur with resultant shallowing of the anterior chamber, corneal touch, and corneal decompensation requiring immediate surgical intervention.

Macular Displacement and Fold

Occasionally following scleral buckling surgery employing an intravitreal air or gas bubble and a highly bullous retinal detachment, the macula may be heterotopically displaced due to shortening of sclera. In some instances the fold may course directly through the fovea, causing distortion, vision loss, or monocular diplopia. This complication can be avoided by minimizing scleral shortening and maximizing subretinal fluid drainage during surgery. Foveal displacement symptoms may be ameliorated by the use of prisms. In severe cases, or when a frank fold is present, if the symptoms are disabling, removal of the buckle and redetachment temporarily may be required.

Infectious Complications

Infectious endophthalmitis following scleral buckling and vitrectomy surgery is a very uncommon complication and almost invariably, in my experience, the result of intravitreal injection in the phakic nonvitrectomized eye as a postoperative maneuver. As a result, great pains should be taken to use sterile technique, including the administration of pre- and postinjection topical antibiotics, when administering or supplementing gas intraoperatively or postoperatively. Treatment of endophthalmitis must be considered an extreme ophthalmic emergency and must include vitreous aspiration for culture and injection of intravitreal antibiotics, with or without vitrectomy.

Although scleral implant and explant material may occasionally become infected (1–4% of cases), this invariably occurs later in the postoperative period (6 weeks up to 20 years). Rarely, a scleral abscess may occur in the immediate postoperative period, heralded by the development of severe ocular pain, orbital swelling out of proportion to the surgical procedure, and purulent discharge. Appropriate therapy for this disorder includes prompt diagnosis, removal of the buckling material, intraoperative orbital and scleral antibiotic lavage, and high-dose intravenous antibiotic therapy after appropriate culture and sensitivity studies have been performed.

Lid Swelling

Lid swelling following scleral buckling occurs frequently enough to be considered an expected phenomenon rather than a true complication. Nonetheless, it is a source of discomfort to the patient and may cause ptosis and limitation of extraocular movement. The incidence and severity of the swelling can be reduced by choosing appropriately sized buckling material, atraumatic surgical technique, and possible use of solid rather than bulky silicone sponge explant material. Orbital swelling is exacerbated by prone positioning (required for patients with intraocular gas bubbles). Ice packs can be used to treat the swelling; systemic steroids are reserved for severe cases.

When lid swelling is severe, or accompanied by signs of severe orbital inflammation including tenderness and redness, the possibility of scleral abscess or a buckle infection should be considered.

Muscle Imbalance

Mild paresis of the extraocular muscles is a common phenomenon during the first 24–72 hours after scleral buckling surgery, particularly when large explants are used, or there has been extensive dissection or revision of buckling material. The use of long-acting local anesthetics for retinal detachment surgery may also contribute to this problem. Motility almost invariably returns to normal within 2 weeks after surgery and symptomatic diplopia can be treated in the intervening time by patching. Up to 5% of patients may have some degree of permanent muscle dysfunction, usually correctable with prisms. The likelihood of this complication is increased by the temporary disinsertion of muscles during scleral buckling, a technique that is rarely indicated. In cases of prolonged motility imbalance, which are uncommon, buckle removal or muscle surgery may be required with or without prism therapy.

Late Postoperative Complications

Infection or Erosion of Implant

The principal late complication of scleral buckling is infection of the implant or explant associated with the development of a fistulous tract. This complication is often heralded by the development of ocular pain, tenderness to palpation over the buckle, conjunctival injection, and lid crusting of a mucoid or frequently purulent nature. This is especially noticeable to the patient upon awakening in the morning. The clinician may determine the site of infection by palpating the globe through the lids, and identifying the tender area. Occasionally, a fistulous tract may develop in the absence of frank clinical infection, although it should be assumed for all practical purposes that the development of a fistula signifies the development of a clinical buckle infection. The likelihood of this complication is increased by poor lid hygiene, possibly the use of sponge rather than solid silicone buckling material, and failure to soak the buckling material intraoperatively (prior to insertion) in an antibiotic solution such as fortified cefazolin or Neosporin. Meticulous closure of Tenon's capsule and conjunctiva and irrigation of the subconjunctival space prior to closure with a topical antibiotic may also reduce the frequency of this complication. Once the patient shows signs and symptoms of an infected explant, removal of the explant is almost always inevitable. In instances in which the buckle has been present for less than 6 weeks and the severity of ocular inflammation is mild, serious consideration should be given to conservative therapy with topical and/or oral antibiotic coverage as well as meticulous lid hygiene to allow formation of a mature chorioretinal adhesion that will maintain retinal reattachment after buckle removal. In the majority of cases, removal of the buckling material is not accompanied by retinal redetachment after this time, provided that all the retinal breaks have been sealed by a thermal modality and there is not extensive residual vitreoretinal traction. I favor supplemental photocoagulation to areas of retinal breaks and/or vitreoretinal traction in instances where the buckle must be removed approximately 1–2 weeks prior to buckle removal.

In some cases, erosion of the conjunctiva and Tenon's capsule tissue overlying the buckle may occur without other clinical signs of infection such as mucopurulent discharge or conjunctival injection. In such cases, a culture should be taken to ascertain that there is no evidence of a conjunctival infection. In some instances, the situation may be stabilized by placement of a homologous scleral or pericardial patch graft over the exposed buckle, over which conjunctiva is then reclosed with an absorbable suture after the edges are trimmed. It can be categorically stated that once a fistulous tract or area of erosion has occurred, reclosing the conjunctiva in that area without placement of additional homologous tissue either in the form of scleral patch graft or autologous donor conjunctiva is

likely to be unsuccessful. Most buckle infections are caused by staphylococcal species and tend to run an indolent course. Occasionally gram-negative infections (including Pseudomonas) produce a more fulminant picture and may be associated with the development of scleral ectasia and frank staphyloma beneath the buckling material. Great care should be exercised in removing buckles in such areas because of the risk of accidental perforation, especially in cases of gram-negative infection. It is also important to remove scleral sutures from all quadrants at the time of buckle removal, since they may contribute to the persistence of infection.

Other Late Complications

A multitude of other complications may occur that are beyond the scope of this chapter. These include development of proliferative changes of the vitreous as manifest by macular pucker or PVR. In general, the likelihood of these complications is increased by any of the other intraoperative or early postoperative complications including scleral perforation, subretinal hemorrhage, choroidal detachment, and fibrinoid syndrome. The reader is advised to consult the chapter on vitrectomy in this and other excellent books on vitrectomy methods for the surgical management of these proliferative complications.

Postoperative Management Techniques

Fluid-Gas Exchange

Fluid-gas exchange is an extremely valuable technique that is applicable to eyes that have previously undergone vitrectomy with the following indications: residual or recurrent subretinal fluid accumulation; persistent intraocular media opacity; evidence of severe intraocular inflammation as manifest by a massive protein deposition (with or without fibrin) in the ocular compartment; to facilitate or prolong intraocular tamponade in eyes with appropriate indications (large retinal tears, proliferative vitreoretinopathy, and occasionally unresolved vitreoretinal traction). Fluid-gas exchange can be performed at the bedside or in a minor surgical suite with either topical or retrobulbar anesthesia, although the latter is recommended in phakic and most pseudophakic patients. Following instillation of topical anesthesia, conjunctival surfaces are prepared with several drops of povidone-iodine (5%) and/or topical antibiotic solution. A lightweight wire speculum is then inserted and the patient rotated into the prone position if aphakic, or the lateral decubitus position with the temporal aspect of the eye to be treated down if phakic or pseudophakic. Fluid-gas exchange is performed with a 10-cc syringe and a short 26- or 27-gauge needle. Sterile air, sulfur hexafluoride (SF6) gas, or perfluoropropane (PFP) is drawn up into the syringe through a 0.22-mm sterile filter. The gas mixture is then diluted to the appropriate concentration through the filter and the plunger of the syringe ultimately returned to the 8-cc marking on the barrel to allow for adequate excursion of the plunger during the first phase of the exchange, which is initiated by withdrawal.

In phakic or pseudophakic patients, the needle is introduced into the vitreous cavity via the temporal pars plana 4 mm, posterior to the limbus, which is in the dependent position with the patient in the lateral decubitus position. The needle tip is brought into view in the midvitreous cavity well clear of the lens and withdrawal initiated. Incremental exchange of 0.5–1.0 ml of fluid is made followed by incremental injections of a similar volume of air or gas leaving the plunger of the syringe in the most dependent position (Figure 10-1). This has the effect of causing fluid to sink gravitationally toward the dependent plunger while keeping air or gas near the hub where it can be continually introduced without the creation of "fish eggs." Care is taken not to incarcerate residual vitreous base by reducing suction as the needle is slowly withdrawn inferiorly during the final stages of phakic exchange (Figure 10-2).

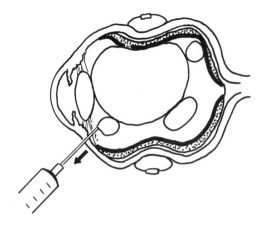

Figure 10-2. Later phase of Figure 10-1. Note lateral decubitus position.

In aphakic patients, the needle is introduced through the nasal or temporal limbus with the dominant hand, depending on which eye is being exchanged, and brought into the midpupillary plane. A similar sequence of small withdrawals and injections is completed until fluid equal in volume to the gas to be injected has been evacuated from the eye and replaced by air or gas (Figure 10-3). Remaining intraocular fluid can be aspirated from the anterior chamber by gently redirecting the needle anteriorly at the end of the procedure (Figure 10-4). IOP at the termination of the exchange should be left in the low-normal range in any eye in which expansile gas is used.

The distinction should be made between the use of expansile gas in general, and the use of an

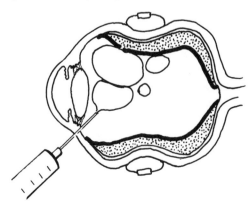

Figure 10-1. Injection of air or gas in phakic previously vitrectomized eye via pars plana.

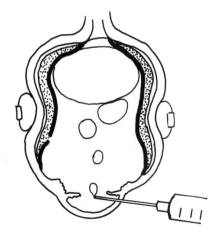

Figure 10-3. Injection of air or gas in aphakic previously vitrectomized eye via limbus. Note prone position.

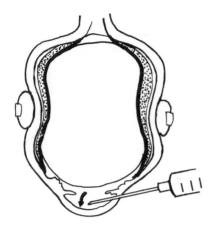

Figure 10-4. Later phase of Figure 10-3. Note face-down position that facilitates complete removal of intraocular fluid.

mitogenic blood retinal breakdown products (which favor the development of postoperative re-proliferation) into the intraocular compartment. Our previous studies indicate that when fluid-gas exchange is performed in eyes with recurrent, subtotal, or total detachment of the retina, 80–85% of patients will demonstrate total or near total reattachment within 24 hours after exchange, with 70% of retinas remaining totally or mostly reattached at 6 months. The long-term results of retinal reattachment in this circumstance appear to be favorably influenced by supplemental photocoagulation through the gas bubble.

Intravitreal Gas Injection

In patients who have not undergone vitrectomy, intravitreal gas may be used for recurrent or residual subretinal fluid, or for extended internal tamponade, although a different technique must be used, and a total gas fill cannot be achieved safely. The risk of intraocular infection appears to be substantially greater in phakic nonvitrectomized patients than in the previous group and, hence, additional caution should be exercised in performing this technique. In contrast to fluid-gas exchange, intravitreal gas injection is generally performed using expansile concentrations of expansile gas, generally 100% SF_6 or PFP, since only small quantities can be injected in the absence of a concomitant release of vitreous fluid.

The technique is virtually the same as that described in Chapter 5. The patient is positioned either supine or in the sitting position with support behind the head and neck. Retrobulbar anesthesia is recommended for instillation of the gas via the pars plana. The lids are separated with a lightweight wire speculum and topical anesthesia and povidone-iodine 5% and topical antibiotics are administered prior to the injection of the gas, which is performed under indirect ophthalmoscopic control to avoid accidental damage to either the lens or detached retina. Premedication with topical IOP lowering medications, osmoglyn, or oral acetazolamide (250 mg) 1 hour prior to the injection and mild digital massage prior to injection are helpful in reducing the severity of the IOP rise immediately after injection. Either 0.3 or 0.4 cc of intravitreal gas is injected, with attempts made to produce a single gas

expansile concentration of an expansile gas. The concentration of 20% (SF_6) and 14% PFP are nonexpansile concentrations of expansile gases; hence no severe increases in IOP should be anticipated although the IOP can be measured in such eyes 4–8 hours after exchange to exclude this potentially catastrophic complication. In some cases, it is advantageous to use an expansile concentration of an expansile gas such as 30–50% SF_6, or 20–25% PFP. This is particularly true in eyes with a large amount of subretinal fluid or eyes in which a total fluid-gas exchange cannot be performed. In these instances, it is especially critical that the closing intraocular pressure be left in the low-normal to soft range; IOP measurements in the first 6–12 hours after injection can avoid major problems. Pressure rises with expansile concentrations of expansile gas can be unpredictable and severe, hence due caution must be exercised. This complication is particularly troublesome in eyes in which an encircling scleral buckle has been applied immediately prior to the fluid-gas exchange, in patients who received nitrous oxide anesthesia (without adequate washout), and in eyes with preexisting rubeosis or open or closed angle glaucoma. In such circumstances, the use of an expansile concentration of gas is strongly discouraged.

When an expansile concentration is used, I currently favor the use of 30% SF_6 or 20% PFP, although the patient must be advised that a subsequent aspiration of gas may be required. These concentrations can help to provide tamponade of inferior retinal breaks and minimize leakage of bubble by a smooth uniform movement, leaving the tip of the needle in the already partially injected gas bubble to reduce the likelihood of "fish eggs." Depending on the desired longevity of the gas bubble as well as the maximal degree of expansion, either SF_6 (two and one-half times expansion), or PFP (four times expansion) may be used. As a general rule, postoperative injection of air is not recommended because of the volume limits imposed. Immediately following injection of gas, the IOP may be elevated in excess of 50 mm Hg and associated with pulsation (and in some cases closure) of the central retinal artery.

I generally perform paracenteses immediately following gas injections to normalize the pressure to approximately 30 mm Hg or less, using full perfusion of the optic nerve as a clinical endpoint. Paracentesis can be dangerous in aphakic and pseudophakic eyes if the posterior capsule is not intact.

Following gas injection, the fundus should be inspected to ascertain that the optic nerve is well perfused and that no gas bubbles have migrated into the subretinal space. The likelihood of this complication can be reduced by avoiding gas injection in eyes with very large open tears, and positioning the head prior to injection in such a way that the large tears are in a dependent position relative to the site of the gas injection.

Previous studies in humans and experimental animals indicate that the injection of a 0.3–0.4 cc volume of expansile intraocular gas is well tolerated, with normalization of the IOP within 40 minutes after injection and no appreciable rise during the period of maximal expansion. In patients with preexisting glaucoma or the recent placement of an encircling buckle, IOP may rise unpredictably and additional caution is thus warranted.

Suggested Reading

Aaberg TM, Pawlowski GJ. Exudative retinal detachments following scleral buckling with cryotherapy. *Am J Ophthalmol* 1972;74:245.

Blumenkranz MS. Management of complicated retinal detachment. In: Tso M, ed. *Retinal Diseases.* Philadelphia: JB Lippincott; 1985.

Blumenkranz MS, Gardner T, Blankenship G. Fluid gas exchange after vitrectomy. I. Indications, technique and results. *Arch Ophthalmol* 1986;104:291.

Charles S. *Vitreous Microsurgery.* 8th Ed. Baltimore: Williams & Wilkins; 1987:207–214.

Chignell A. *Retinal Detachment Surgery.* Berlin/Heidelberg/New York: Springer-Verlag; 1980:139–162.

Fison PN, Chignell AH. Diplopia after retinal detachment surgery. *Br J Ophthalmol* 1987;71(7):521–525.

Grizzard WS, Hilton GF, Hammer ME, Taren D. A multivariate analysis of anatomic success of retinal detachments treated with scleral buckling. *Graefes Arch Clin Exp Ophthalmol* 1994;232(1):1–7.

Hay A, Flynn HW Jr., Hoffman JI, Rivera AH. Needle penetration of the globe during retrobulbar and peribulbar injections. *Ophthalmology* 1991;98(7):1017–1024.

Kanski J. *Retinal Detachment: A Colour Manual of Diagnosis and Treatment.* Oxford: Butterworth; 1986:129–154.

Levkovitch-Verbin H, Treister G, Moisseiev J. Pneumatic retinopexy as supplemental therapy for persistent retinal detachment after scleral buckling operation. *Acta Ophthalmol Scand* 1998;76(3):353–355.

Maeno T, Maeda N, Ikeda T, Tano Y. Tissue plasminogen activator treatment of postvitrectomy pupillary fibrin membrane. *Nippon Ganka Gakkai Zasshi* 1991;95(11): 1124–1128.

Packer A, Maggiano J, Aaberg T, et al. Serous choroidal detachment after retinal detachment surgery. *Arch Ophthalmol* 1983;101:1221.

Regillo CD, Benson WE. *Retinal Detachment: Diagnosis and Management*, 3rd Ed. Philadelphia: Lippincott-Raven; 1998.

Schepens C. *Retinal Detachment and Allied Diseases.* Vol. 1. Philadelphia: WB Saunders; 1983:1024–1086.

Tabandeh H, Flaxel C, Sullivan PM, Leaver PK, Flynn HW Jr, Schiffman J. Scleral rupture during retinal detachment surgery: risk factors, management options, and outcomes. *Ophthalmology* May 2000;107(5):848–852.

van Meurs JC, Humalda D, Mertens DA, Peperkamp E. Retinal folds through the macula. *Doc Ophthalmol* 1991;78(3–4):335–340.

Wade E, Flynn HW Jr, Olsen KR, Blumenkranz MS, Nicholson D. Subretinal hemorrhage management by pars plana vitrectomy and internal drainage. *Arch Ophthalmol* 1990;108:973–978.

Wilkenson CP, Rice TA. *Michels Retinal Detachment*, 2nd ed. Philadelphia: Mosby; 1997.

Index

Note: Page numbers followed by "t" indicate tables; page numbers followed by "f" indicate figures.

Adjuvant therapy, in macular hole surgery, 112–113
Anesthesia
    agents, 48–49
    anatomic considerations, 44–48
    general
        description of, 43, 53–54
        local anesthesia and, 54
    local
        complications of, 51, 53
        description of, 43, 48
        general anesthesia and, 54
        technique for, 50–51, 52f
    minimal, 54
    monitoring during, 50
    needles, 49–50
    patient selection considerations, 43–44, 44t
    pharmacologic considerations, 48–49
    premedication agents, 50
    techniques
        Atkinson, 43, 47–48, 48f
        local, 50–51, 52f
        retrobulbar injection, 50, 52f
Annulus of Zinn, 45
Aphakia, retinal detachment associated with, 25
Atkinson technique, 43, 47–48, 48f
Atrophic retina, 9
Autologous serum, 113
a-wave (ERG), 19–20

Biomicroscopy, fundal examination using, 9
Breaks. *See* Retinal breaks
Bruch's membrane, 2f
Bupivacaine
    advantages and disadvantages of, 51t
    description of, 43, 48

    dosing of, 49t
    lidocaine and, 51t
b-wave (ERG), 19–20, 20f

Carbonic anhydrase inhibitors, 38
Cataracts, macular hole surgery as cause of, 115
Central retinal artery occlusion, 21
Central retinal vein occlusion, 21
Choriocapillaris, 1, 2f
Chorioretinal pigmentation, 7
Choroid
    anatomy of, 2f
    detachment of
        echographic imaging of, 17
        hemorrhagic, 17, 18f
        scleral buckling as cause, 123–124
        serous, 17
Circumferential traction lines, 7
Complications, of vitreoretinal surgery
    anterior segment ischemia, 124
    cataract, 124
    choroidal detachment, 123–124
    classification of, 119
    description of, 119
    exudative retinal detachment, 123
    eyelid swelling, 125
    fibrinoid reaction, 124
    globe rupture, 120
    infections, 125
    macular displacement and fold, 125
    muscle imbalance, 125
    ocular hypertension, 121–123
    postoperative management of
        fluid-gas exchange, 126–128
        intravitreal gas injection, 128–129

Complications, of vitreoretinal surgery *(continued)*
  retinal folds, 122
  retinal incarceration in sclerotomy site,
    102–103, 120–121
  scleral suture penetration, 119–120
  subretinal hemorrhage, 121
Conjunctiva, 6
Contact lens examination, 9
Corneal erosions, 103
Cryopexy
  advantages of, 27
  complications associated with, 27–28
  description of, 27
  disadvantages of, 27
  laser photocoagulation vs., comparisons
    between, 28–29
  for retinal incarceration, 120
  technique, 29–30
c-wave (ERG), 19–20
Cyclopentolate hydrochloride, 6

Diabetic retinopathy
  description of, 69
  membrane removal
    indications, 98
    surgical technique, 98–100
  silicone oil for, 95
  vitrectomy for, 99f
Duranest. *See* Etidocaine

Echography
  A-scan, 12
  B-scan, 11–12
  diagnostic and evaluative uses of
    choroidal detachment, 17
    foreign bodies, 17–18, 19f
    posterior segment, 12
    retinal detachment
      closed-funnel, 13, 14f
      diabetic tractional, 13, 15f
      nonrhegmatogenous, 15–17
      open-funnel, 13, 14f
      rhegmatogenous, 12–13
      trauma, 17–18
  history of, 11
Ehlers-Danlos syndrome, 26
Electrophysiology
  description of, 18
  electroretinogram. *See* Electroretinogram
  visually evoked potential, 21–22
Electroretinogram
  bright-flash, 19–21
  description of, 19–21, 20f
  diagnostic and evaluative uses

central retinal artery occlusion, 21
central retinal vein occlusion, 21
partial retinal detachment, 21
proliferative diabetic retinopathy, 21
Endophthalmitis
  after scleral buckling, 125
  vitrectomy for, 70
Epinephrine, 49
Epiretinal membranes
  description of, 85–86
  macular, 69–70, 110
  membrane peeling for. *See* Membrane peeling
  removal of, during macular hole surgery, 110
Ethmoidal nerve, 46f
Etidocaine, 48, 49t
Explants, for scleral buckling
  description of, 5
  infections in, 124
  selection of, 60
  silicone bands, 60, 60f
External limiting membrane, 2f
Eyelids
  evaluation of, 6
  swelling of, after scleral buckling, 125

Fibrinoid reaction, 124
Fluid-gas exchange, 126–128
Forceps, 73f
Foreign bodies, 17–18, 19f
Fovea
  description of, 1
  limited translocation of, 101
Frontal nerve, 45
Fundus
  examination of, 6–9
  peripheral changes in, 9
  scleral buckling evaluations, 67

Ganglion layer, 2f
Gas injections
  fluid-gas exchange, 126–128
  intravitreal, 128–129
  for scleral buckling, 68
  tamponade use. *See* Intraocular tamponade
General anesthesia
  description of, 43, 53–54
  local anesthesia and, 54
Giant retinal tear
  definition of, 96
  treatment of
    perfluorocarbon liquid, 95–96
    silicone oil, 95
    surgical, 96–98

Glaucoma, 96

Hemorrhage
    retinal, 9
    subretinal. *See* Subretinal hemorrhage
    surgical onset of, 103
Hyaluronidase, 49

Indirect ophthalmoscopy
    fundal examination using, 6–7
    retinal breaks detected using, 24
    subretinal fluid drainage, 66–67
    technique for, 6
Informed consent, 10
Infraorbital nerve, 46f–47f
Infratrochlear nerve, 47f
Inner limiting membrane
    anatomy of, 2f
    removal during macular hole surgery, 110, 111f
Inner nuclear layer, 2f
Inner plexiform layer, 2f
Intraocular pressure, increased
    in macular hole surgery, 114
    ocular hypertension secondary to, 121–122
    in scleral buckling, 56
Intraocular tamponade
    gases
        description of, 112, 114
        indications, 94
        ocular hypertension caused by, 95
        perfluoropropane, 94, 127–128
        sulfur hexafluoride, 94, 127
        types of, 94
        vitrectomy use, 94–95
    for macular hole surgery, 105, 112
    for retinal detachments, 103
    for scleral buckling, 68
    silicone oil, 112
Intravitreal gas injection, 128–129

Lacrimal nerve, 45, 46f–47f
Laser photocoagulation
    advantages of, 28
    cryopexy vs., comparisons between, 28–29
    description of, 28
    disadvantages of, 28
    for pneumatic retinopexy, 35, 37f
    posterior retinal break treated using, 90f
    technique, 30–31
    wavelength setting, 28
Lattice degeneration
    description of, 7
    retinal detachment risks, 26

Lens
    subluxation of, 6
    vitrectomy-induced damage, 103
Lensectomy, 83–85
Lidocaine
    advantages and disadvantages of, 51t
    bupivacaine and, 51t
    complications associated with, 53
    description of, 49t
    dosing of, 49t
Lids. *See* Eyelids
Local anesthesia
    complications of, 51, 53
    description of, 43, 48
    general anesthesia and, 54
    technique for, 50–51, 52f

Macula
    anatomy of, 1
    displacement of, after scleral buckling, 125
Macular hole
    classification of, 106t
    clinical findings, 107f
    differential diagnosis, 106
    surgery for
        case selection, 106
        cataract formation after, 113
        complications associated with, 114–115,
            115t
        goals of, 105, 116
        indications, 105–106
        instrumentation, 108t
        patient positioning after, 113–114
        postoperative care, 113–114
        preoperative evaluation, 106, 108
        prognostic factors, 106, 106t
        success rates, 107f
        summary overview of, 115–116
        technique
            adjuvants, 112–113
            air-fluid exchange, 111–112
            epiretinal membrane removal, 110
            internal limiting membrane removal, 110,
                111f
            tamponade, 112, 114
            vitrectomy, 108–110
    techniques for assessing, 106, 108
    traumatic, 106
Marcaine. *See* Bupivacaine
Marfan's syndrome, 6
Membrane peeling
    epiretinal membrane
        with attached retina, 86
        with retinal detachment, 86–88

Membrane peeling *(continued)*
  indications, 85–86
  instrumentation, 86
  peripheral membrane, 88
  retinal breaks during, 103
  technique, 86–89
Membranes
  epiretinal. *See* Epiretinal membranes
  inner limiting
    anatomy of, 2f
    removal during macular hole surgery, 110,
      111f
  peeling of. *See* Membrane peeling
  peripheral, 88
  removal of
    in diabetic retinopathy, 98–100
    in macular hole surgery, 110, 111f
  subfoveal neovascular
    description of, 70
    surgical removal of, 100–101
Miosis, 26, 67
Muscle cone, 44–45
Myopia, retinal detachment risks associated with,
    25–26

Nasociliary nerve, 45, 46f
Needles, for retrobulbar anesthesia, 49–50
Nerve(s)
  ciliary, 3f
  ethmoidal, 46f
  frontal, 45
  infraorbital, 46f–47f
  infratrochlear, 47f
  lacrimal, 45, 47f
  nasociliary, 45, 46f
  oculomotor, 47
  optic, 45
  supraorbital, 45, 46f–47f
  supratrochlear, 45, 47f
  trigeminal, 45
  zygomatic, 46f–47f
  zygomaticofacial, 46f
  zygomaticotemporal, 46f–47f

Ocular coherence tomography, for macular hole
    evaluations, 108
Ocular examination
  in retinal detachment patient, 5–6
  in vitrectomy patient, 72–74
Ocular histoplasmosis syndrome, 100
Ocular hypertension, 95, 103, 121–123
Oculomotor nerve, 47
Ophthalmic artery, 45

Ophthalmoscopy. *See* Indirect ophthalmoscopy
Optic canal, 45
Optic foramen, 45
Optic nerve, 45
Orbit, anterior, 44
Outer nuclear layer, 2f
Outer plexiform layer, 2f

Panfunduscopic lenses, 9
Pars plana vitrectomy, 11
Perfluorocarbon liquid
  giant retinal tears treated using, 95–98
  proliferative vitreoretinopathy treated using,
    91–92
  during vitrectomy, 81
Perfluoropropane, 94, 127–128
Peripheral membrane, 88
Peripheral retinal dialysis, 102
Phakic retinal detachment, 25
Phenylephrine hydrochloride, 6
Photocoagulation. *See* Laser photocoagulation
Photoreceptors, 1
Platelet concentrates, 113
Pneumatic retinopexy
  bubble
    characteristics of, 34–35
    complications associated with, 40
    mechanism of action, 33
    perfluoropropane, 34
    selection of, 34–35
  complications of, 40
  history of, 33
  mechanism of action, 33
  patient selection, 33–34
  phakic status and, 40
  postoperative care, 38–39
  scleral buckling vs., comparisons between, 41
  success criteria, 40–41
  technique
    antibiotic use, 37–38
    laser photocoagulation, 35, 37f
    steamroller, 37–38, 39f
    summary overview of, 36t
Posterior segment vitrectomy. *See* Vitrectomy
Posterior uveal melanoma
  echographic imaging of, 16, 16f
  retinal detachment vs., 16
Posterior vitreous detachment
  description of, 3
  echographic imaging of, 13–14
  surgical methods for creating, in macular hole
    surgery, 109
  total retinal detachment vs., 13–14

Posterior vitreous separation, 3, 4f
Proliferative diabetic retinopathy, 21
　vitrectomy for, 98–100
Proliferative vitreoretinopathy
　anterior, 13, 15f
　treatment of
　　perfluorocarbon liquid, 91f
　　pneumatic retinopexy, 34
　　silicone oil, 95–96
Proparacaine, 9
Pseudophakia, 25
Pulse oximeter, for anesthesia monitoring, 50

Radial sponges, 63
Rectus muscles, 47
Relaxing retinotomies
　indications, 92
　technique, 92–94
Retina
　anatomy of, 1–3, 2f
　folds, 122
　hemorrhage of, 9
　incarceration in sclerotomy site, 102–103,
　　120–121
　translocation of, 101
Retinal breaks
　asymptomatic, 23
　atrophic, 25
　classification of, 26
　definition of, 3–4
　detection of, 10, 23–24, 58–59
　fellow eyes, 26
　indirect ophthalmoscopy evaluations, 6, 24, 58
　lesions that simulate, 9
　macular hole surgery as cause of, 114
　membrane peeling-induced, 103
　operculated, 4, 25
　subretinal fluid and, treatment decisions
　　regarding
　　cryopexy, 30
　　decision-making criteria, 26
　　laser photocoagulation, 31
　symptoms of, 23–24
　tractional, 25
　treatment of
　　cryopexy. *See* Cryopexy
　　decisions regarding, 24–27
　　follow-up care, 31–32
　　laser photocoagulation. *See* Laser photoco-
　　　agulation
　　success rate, 31
　　during vitrectomy, 89–90
　vitrectomy-induced, 103
　without scleral depression, 7

Retinal detachment
　in aphakic patient, 25
　closed-funnel, 13, 14f
　diabetic tractional, 13, 15f
　electroretinogram evaluations of, 21
　epiretinal membrane with, 86–88
　exudative, 123
　factors that cause, 4
　in fellow eyes, 26
　incidence of, 24
　Lincoff's rules, 9–10
　myopia and, 25–26
　open-funnel, 13, 14f
　in phakic patient, 25
　pneumatic retinopexy for, 34
　preoperative evaluations
　　description of, 5
　　fundal examination, 6–9
　　history-taking, 5
　　informed consent, 10
　　ocular examination, 5–6
　　retinal breaks, 9
　rhegmatogenous
　　description of, 1, 55
　　macular hole surgery as cause of, 114
　serous, 17
　vitrectomy for. *See* Vitrectomy
Retinal pigment epithelium
　anatomy of, 1–3, 2f
　description of, 1
　macular hole surgery effects, 115
　retina attachment to, 4
Retinal tears. *See* Giant retinal tear; Retinal breaks
Retinal tufts, 9
Retinectomy, 93–94
Retinopathy of prematurity, 70
Retinoschisis
　acquired, 9
　atrophic retina vs., 9
　congenital, 9
Retrobulbar injection
　complications associated with, 53
　technique, 50, 52f
RPE. *See* Retinal pigment epithelium

Scissors, 72f
Sclera, 1, 3
Scleral buckling
　anesthesia, 44, 56
　complications of
　　choroidal detachment, 123–124
　　exudative retinal detachment, 119–120
　　eyelid swelling, 125
　　fibrinoid reaction, 124

Scleral buckling, complications of *(continued)*
    macular displacement and fold, 125
    penetration with scleral sutures, 119–120
  cryopexy use, 59–60
  description of, 55
  explant selection, 5, 60–64, 124
  gas injections, 68
  intraocular pressure concerns, 56
  intrascleral suture placement, 64–65
  laser photocoagulation use, 60
  opening conjunctiva, 56–58
  pneumatic retinopexy vs., comparisons
    between, 41
  preoperative management, 55–56
  retinal break localization, 58–59
  retinal detachment categorization for, 55–56
  subretinal fluid drainage, 61, 65–68
  sutures, 64–65
  vitrectomy and, 90
Scleral implant
  description of, 5
  erosion of, 125–126
  infections in, 124–126
Sclerotomy
  for lensectomy, 84
  for vitrectomy, 76–78
Silicone oil
  complications associated with, 96
  description of, 95
  indications, 95–96
  injection techniques for, 96
  tamponade uses, 112
Slit-lamp examination
  in retinal detachment patient, 6
  in vitrectomy patient, 72
Stickler's syndrome, 26
Subfoveal neovascular membranes, surgical
    removal of, 100–101
Subretinal fluid
  drainage of
    complications associated with
      retinal folds, 122
      subretinal hemorrhage, 121
    inability to complete successfully, 120
    persistence of fluid after
      description of, 122–123
      intravitreal gas injection for, 128–129
    in scleral buckling, 61, 65–68
  retinal breaks and, treatment decisions regarding
    cryopexy, 30
    decision-making criteria, 26
    laser photocoagulation, 31
  retinal detachment accumulation of, 10

Subretinal hemorrhage
  disciform scar, 15f
  echographic imaging of, 13, 15f
  predisposing factors, 121
  during subretinal fluid drainage, 121
Subretinal space
  echography evaluations of, 13
  in retinal detachment, 13
Sulfur hexafluoride, 94, 127
Suprachoroidal hemorrhage, 17
Supraorbital nerve, 45, 46f–47f
Supratrochlear nerve, 45, 47f
Surgery. *See specific surgery*

Tamponade. *See* Intraocular tamponade
Tenon's space, 56, 57f, 126
Tissue manipulator, 72f
Transforming growth factor–beta, 113
Trauma
  echographic evaluations of, 17–18, 19f
  macular holes caused by, 106
  vitrectomy for, 70
Trigeminal nerve, 45

VEP. *See* Visually evoked potential
Visual field evaluation, 5–6
Visually evoked potential, 21–22
Vitrectomy
  anesthesia, 44, 74
  complications of, 102–103
  diabetic retinopathy treated using, 98–100, 99f
  fluid-gas exchange after, 126–128
  giant retinal tear, 96–98
  goals of, 69, 69t
  indications, 69–71
  instrumentation
    arranging of, 74, 75f
    types of, 71, 72f–73f
  intraocular gases used during, 94–95
  intraocular infusion solutions, 75–76
  lensectomy, 83–85
  in macular hole surgery, 108–110
  membrane peeling
    with attached retina, 86
    indications, 85–86
    instrumentation, 86
    peripheral membrane, 88
    with retinal detachment, 86–88
    technique, 86–89
  ocular examination before, 72–74
  ocular histoplasmosis syndrome treated using, 100
  patient preparation for, 74

perfluorocarbon liquid, 91–92
relaxing retinotomies, 92–94
retinal breaks treated during, 89–90
retinal detachment treated during, 90
retinectomy during, 93–94
scleral buckling during, 90
silicone oil use, 95–96
subfoveal neovascular membrane removal,
    100–101
surgical planning for, 74
technique
    description of, 78–83
    entrance into the eye, 76–78
    incisions, 76
    perfluorocarbon liquid, 81
    posterior hyaloid incision, 79–80
    posterior vitreous removal, 79–80
    sclerotomy, 76–78
    suturing, 83
    vitreous separation, 81–82

Vitreoretinal forceps, 73f
Vitreoretinal scissors, 72f
Vitreous
    anatomy of, 3–4
    incarceration in sclerotomy site, during vitrec-
        tomy, 102–103
    separation of, 3
Vortex veins, 1, 3f

Watzke-Allen test, 108
Wydase. *See* Hyaluronidase

Xylocaine. *See* Lidocaine

Zygomatic nerve, 46f–47f
Zygomaticofacial nerve, 46f
Zygomaticotemporal nerve, 46f–47f

From Butterworth-Heinemann Essential Ophthalmic Surgery References

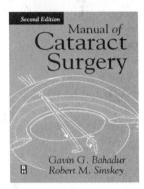

Second Edition
Manual of
Cataract
Surgery

Gavin G. Bahadur
Robert M. Sinskey

1999, 128 pp., Paperback,
0-7506-7082-7, $47.50

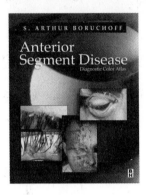

S. ARTHUR BORUCHOFF
Anterior
Segment Disease
Diagnostic Color Atlas

October 2000, 288 pp.,
Hardcover,
0-7506-7181-5, $115.00

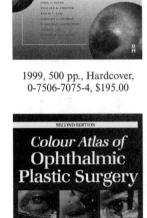

THE UNIVERSITY OF MIAMI
BASCOM PALMER EYE INSTITUTE
Atlas of
Ophthalmology
EDITOR
RICHARD K. PARRISH II

1999, 500 pp., Hardcover,
0-7506-7075-4, $195.00

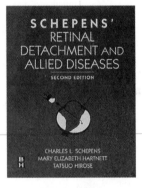

SCHEPENS'
RETINAL
DETACHMENT AND
ALLIED DISEASES
SECOND EDITION

CHARLES L. SCHEPENS
MARY ELIZABETH HARTNETT
TATSUO HIROSE

July 2000, 784 pp.,
Hardcover,
0-7506-9837-3, $275.00

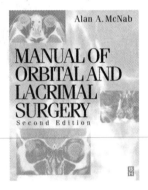

Alan A. McNab
MANUAL OF
ORBITAL AND
LACRIMAL
SURGERY
Second Edition

1998, 160 pp., Paperback,
0-7506-3997-0, $65.00

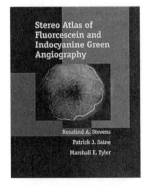

SECOND EDITION
Colour Atlas of
Ophthalmic
Plastic Surgery

A. G. TYERS • J. R. O. COLLIN

January 2001, 368 pp.,
Hardcover, 0-7506-4254-8,
$175.00

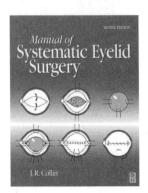

SECOND EDITION
Manual of
Systematic Eyelid
Surgery

J.R. Collin

1999, 184 pp., Paperback,
0-7506-4572-5, $80.00

TO ORDER:

Call: 1-800-366-2665

or

Visit us on the web:
www.bh.com

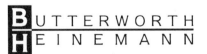

BUTTERWORTH
HEINEMANN

Stereo Atlas of
Fluorescein and
Indocyanine Green
Angiography

Rosalind A. Stevens
Patrick J. Saine
Marshall E. Tyler

1999, 147 pp., Hardcover,
0-7506-7001-0, $90.00